Mrs Celia Bernardo
9400 Aqueduct Ave
North Hills, CA 91343-2038

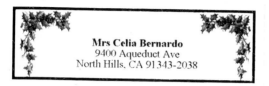

Elizabeth Gross Cohn, RN, CEN, EMT-CC
Staff Nurse
Department of Emergency Medicine
North Shore University Hospital
Manhasset, New York

Mary Gilroy-Doohan, MD, FACEP
Director, Emergency Department
North Shore University Hospital at Glen Cove
Glen Cove, New York

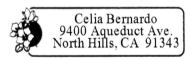

flip and see ECG

W.B. SAUNDERS COMPANY
A Division of Harcourt Brace & Company
Philadelphia London Toronto Montreal Sydney Tokyo

W.B. SAUNDERS COMPANY
A Division of Harcourt Brace & Company

The Curtis Center
Independence Square West
Philadelphia, Pennsylvania 19106

Library of Congress Cataloging-in-Publication Data

Cohn, Elizabeth Gross.
    Flip and see ECG / Elizabeth Gross Cohn and Mary Gilroy-Doohan. —
1st ed.
        p.   cm.
    ISBN 0–7216–5834–2
    1. Electrocardiography—Handbooks, manuals, etc.   I. Gilroy
-Doohan, Mary.   II. Title.
    [DNLM: 1. Electrocardiography.   WG 140 C678f 1996]
    RC683.5.E5C59   1996
616.1´207547—dc20
DNLM/DLC   95-20111

Flip and See ECG   0–7216–5834–2

Printed in the United States of America

Last digit is the print number: 9   8   7   6   5   4   3   2   1

This book is dedicated to

My parents, Ronald and Beatrice Gross,
for all their encouragement and support.
Their effort and faith
made this book possible.

Bruce, Zachary, and Hannah Cohn,
for providing technical and emotional support.

My father-in-law, the late George Cohn,
in the deepest hopes that the information contained here
will help to save the lives of others.

Mr. Joseph Gorski,
who knew exactly what to do, and did it.

The team of professionals at W.B. Saunders:
Amy Norwitz, Bill Donnelly,
Deborah Lynam, Lori Irvine,
Rita Martello

The physicians, nurses, paramedics, and EMTs of the
Emergency Department at North Shore University
Hospital; they are my best teachers and friends.

My wonderful editor, Lisa Biello,
for whom I have the most profound respect and admiration.

Acknowledgments

· ·

I am profoundly grateful to those who took personal time and effort to read rough drafts and check endless strips of rhythms; this book is a tribute to their efforts:

Denise Bellingham
Carol Della Ratta
Mary Anne Dumas
Michael Irise
Susan Irise
Thomas J. Rahilly
Leslie Tyson
Carolyn Willson

A Word From Our Sponsor

··

This book is humbly dedicated to Willem Einthoven, inventor of the electrocardiogram machine.

One hundred and ten years ago, it was recognized that electrical charges were involved with the beating of the heart and that changes in the rhythm of the heart correlated with changes in the electrical patterns. The only known method for recording these cardiac events was by direct contact with the open, exposed heart. These patients usually died.

In 1887, Augustus Waller invented the *electrode*. This device allowed the electrical currents to be measured through *intact skin,* which was a tremendous boon to patients and medical personnel alike. His electrode was a large magnetic plate hooked up to a *capillary electrometer*. This capillary electrometer was a column of mercury that rose and fell with changes in the electrical field. Despite the electrode's ability to monitor electrical impulses through intact skin, it gave inaccurate readings because of a long lag time between the action of the heart and the action of the mercury. Additionally the physician needed to perform a long, laborious mathematical calculation to establish the pattern. This was a good invention, but with the lag time of the mercury and the long math calculation, by the time the measurement was completed the action of the heart was long finished, and sometimes so was the patient.

Willem Einthoven is credited with the invention of the electrocardiograph machine, for which he was awarded the Nobel Prize. The electrocardiogram, the graphic representation of electrical activity, is also known as the *EKG* or *ECG* ("*electrokardiogramm*" from the German, abbreviated EKG). The medical profession currently uses these abbreviations interchangeably.

Einthoven's ECG machine was a fine quartz wire suspended in a magnetic field. When subjected to an electrical current, the wire deflected according to the charge. This motion was magnified and photographed on a moving reel of film. Because it was very light in weight, the wire responded almost instantaneously to any changes in the electrical current. Einthoven established the criteria for normal ECGs and named the waves P, QRS, and T. He further designated the three points on the body where the electrodes should be placed.

Today the ECG machine remains one of the single most important tools in medicine used for diagnosis, monitoring, gauging response to therapy, and recording past events. We rely on ECGs daily in ambulances and hospitals and by phone line to save the lives of thousands.

Physical Examination

....

Obtaining a Patient History

Using an organized approach to obtaining a patient history and physical examination results in a complete and accurate clinical picture. The systems listed here assist practitioners in securing the necessary history and information. Many experienced clinicians start their assessment with how the patient looks. They then ask if there is a past cardiac history. There are more than 25 differential diagnoses* for the chest pain patient. The beginning practitioner should be aware that *acute myocardial infarction,* or heart attack, is among the most critical of the chest pain scenarios. All chest pain should be taken seriously and treated as cardiac until proven otherwise.

AMPLER system

In the *AMPLER* system, the patient is asked about
*A*llergies
*M*edications—especially cardiac medications, antihypertensive drugs, antiarrhythmics, and insulin
*P*ast history—anyone with a history of a cardiac condition and current chest pain is considered to be a cardiac patient
*L*ast meal —necessary information for anesthesia
*E*vents —in the case of chest pain, it is especially noteworthy if the pain woke the patient from sleep or continued when the patient was at rest
*R*isk factors—smoking, diabetes, hypertension, coronary artery disease, and no regular exercise

---

*Angina, acute myocardial infarction, bronchitis, cardiogenic shock, cardiac tamponade, aortic dissection, leaking aortic aneurysm, mitral valve prolapse, aortic stenosis, aortic insufficiency, pericarditis, pericardial effusion, pleurisy, pleural effusion, pneumothorax, pneumomediastinum, pulmonary hypertension, pulmonary embolism, pneumonia, tumors, esophagitis, esophageal spasm, hiatal hernia, gastritis, perforated duodenal ulcer, pancreatitis, cholecystitis, musculoskeletal disorders, rib fractures, and costochondritis, to name some.

The *PQRST* system helps patients to describe chest pain:

Provokes—What makes the pain worse, or better? Does it increase with movement? Stop when you rest? Can you take a deep breath?

Quality —What kind of pain? Is it sharp and stabbing or dull? Does it feel like pressure? Is it intermittent—does it come and go?

Radiates —Does it go anywhere? Jaw? Left arm?

Severity —Rate the pain/pressure on a scale of 1–10, with 1 being very little pain and 10 being very severe. (This is used diagnostically and to gauge efficiency of treatment.)

Time —How long have you had the pain? (In cardiac chest pain, *time is muscle.* The longer the duration of pain, the more damage.)

Vital Signs

Vital signs for assessment include

1. Pulse
2. Blood pressure
3. Respiration—number and effort
4. Lung sounds
5. Skin temperature (diaphoresis?)
6. Chest pain rated on a scale of 1–10
7. Description of pain
8. Cardiac/diabetic history; owing to neuropathy, diabetic patients have "silent myocardial infarctions," heart attacks without chest pain

MOVE

To remember the steps for treatment, use **MOVE**:

Monitor
Oxygen
Venous access
ECG (12-lead)

Contents

· ·

flip and see ECG

"Medic 1—your signal is all broken up; we read nothing but static. What ECG rhythm do you read at your end?"

As my ambulance raced toward the hospital, I stared at the tiny screen with a green line bleeping across it and felt my own heart stop. The doctor at the other end of the Medical Control radio was waiting. Whatever I said would determine the treatment for this patient. He would get medicated, shocked, transported, or pronounced dead, completely based on *my* ability to identify this rhythm correctly.

"Medic 1—this is base; What do you read!?"

Flip and See ECG has three fundamental concepts:

1. **If it walks like a duck, and quacks like a duck, it's a duck.**

2. **Meaning—not memorization.**

3. **Trust yourself.**

How to Approach ECGs

1. IF IT WALKS LIKE A DUCK, AND QUACKS LIKE A DUCK, IT'S A DUCK

This manual will enable you to learn the basics of 3-lead ECG interpretation so you can start *immediately*. Its focus is on teaching you the most important and frequently encountered rhythms. Later, you can master the subtle distinctions that become important for more advanced ECG monitor interpretation. While not wanting to offend purists, this book leans in the direction of simplifying concepts whenever possible and not distracting the learner with every conceivable outcome or variation.

ECG monitor interpretation is a serious medical science. This book and careful practice provide an excellent starting place for those who desire to learn ECG interpretation. It is also helpful to those in need of a basic review.

2. MEANING—NOT MEMORIZATION

You can interpret almost any 3-lead ECG with an understanding of a few basic concepts. The exercises in this book are meant to be done as you go along, open-book style. As in crocheting, after you master a few basic stitches, you can make an entire blanket.

3. TRUST YOURSELF

Relax, and enjoy this book. You *can* read and interpret 3-lead ECGs. Everything you need to know is contained in this handbook. This method has been successfully used to teach classes of nurses, paramedics, and medical students. Based on this success, we tried it on neighbors, friends, parents, and people who have not even been examined by a doctor in 12 years, and they were all confidently reading 3-lead ECG in *less than 2 hours*.

The Heart

LOCATION

The scar that open-heart surgery leaves is a long, vertical, thick red line that runs down the full length of a patient's chest.

I was assigned to obtain an apical pulse on a man who had just been rolled out of surgery. You take an apical pulse by placing your stethoscope directly over the heart and counting the number of beats you hear in 1 minute.

I confidently stepped up to the patient's bedside and lifted his gown. I stared down at this fresh thick, long scar and gray chest hair, shaved from the operation. Now all I needed to do was listen directly over the heart.

I thought that the patient would be sore from having his chest peeled back like the skin of an orange; so I wanted to be especially careful to gently place the bell of my stethoscope directly over the heart, but my hand froze: Where exactly is the heart located?

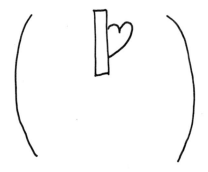

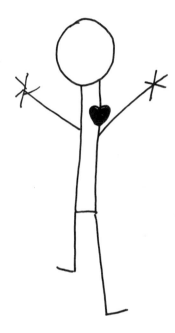

I placed my stethoscope down carefully, about 1 inch below the left nipple and in toward the center (sternum). Quietly I listened to the lub-dub beat of his heart.

The heart lies in the center of the chest, under the sternum and in between the lungs. Two-thirds of it lies to the left of the sternum. It is approximately the size of your fist and weighs about 10.6 oz.

ANATOMY (STRUCTURE)

The heart is divided into four chambers.

The two top chambers are called the atria. The two bottom chambers are called the ventricles. The heart is actually a two-

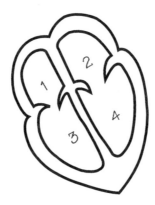

sided pump. The left side pumps oxygenated blood, and the right side pumps deoxygenated blood. When the atria contract, blood is pushed into the ventricles through valves. When the ventricles contract, blood is pumped out into the body and the lungs. The septum is cartilage that separates the two sides of the heart. One-way valves located between the atria and the ventricles keep the blood flow headed in the right direction.

1. Divide the heart into four quadrants.
2. Label the right and left sides.*
3. Label the atria and the ventricles.
4. Draw arrows indicating blood flow from the atria to the ventricles and out to the body and lungs.

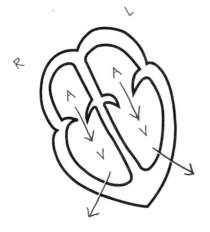

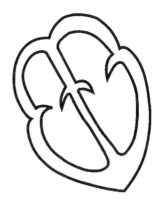

_____

*In medicine, the _anatomical_ position is used to designate the location of body parts. It is the _patient's_ right and left sides.

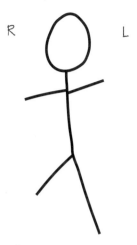

R   L

The anatomical position.

The blood that flows through the heart is the blood used to nourish the body. The heart muscle itself has its own blood supply furnished by the coronary arteries.

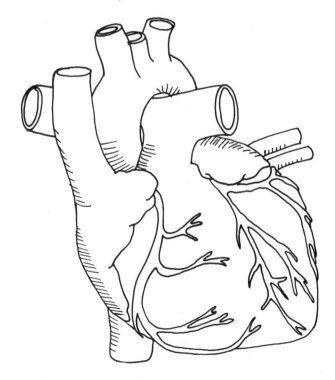

PHYSIOLOGY (FUNCTION)

The function of the heart is to circulate blood to all the tissues of the body. The blood supplies the tissues with oxygen and removes carbon dioxide and waste products. The heart can also be divided into a right and a left side. These two sides expand and contract simultaneously but receive blood flow from two separate areas of the body.

Cardiac Cycle

The cardiac cycle consists of two phases: contraction and relaxation. It is as if you squeezed a sponge in a bowl of water. When the heart contracts, it is squeezing blood out to the body. As the heart relaxes, it is expanding and refilling. These are known as the systolic (the heart squeezing) and the diastolic (the heart relaxing) phases of the cardiac cycle.

The contraction (depolarization) and relaxation (repolarization) of the heart is actually a mechanical process initiated by an electrical "spark." When the heart is resting, the cells are negatively charged inside and positively charged outside. When an electrical impulse is introduced, there is a wave of activity, and the cells become positively charged on the inside and negatively charged on the outside. This action causes the muscle to contract.

Think of it as a "wave" at a baseball game. One person in the bleachers starts the wave by standing up and throwing his or her hands in the air. As the person sits down, the next person stands up, and the next person continues, and the next, until it goes all the way around the stadium.

EXCUSE ME
What does all this have to do with ECGs?

Answer: This electrical activity is what is recorded on the ECG machine. The positive and negative charges are what is actually being picked up by the monitor.

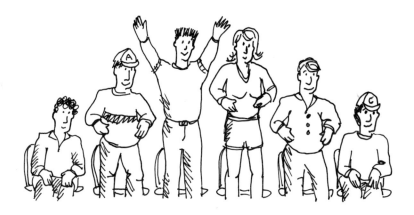

Summary

Let's review: The contraction and relaxation of the heart is a mechanical event prompted by an electrical impulse. When the myocardial cells receive this electrical impulse, the heart depolarizes, changing from a negative charge inside the cells to a positive charge, and the impulse spreads through the muscle, causing the muscle to contract.

The heart cells then repolarize, returning to a negative charge on the inside and a positive charge on the outside, and are now ready for the next stimulus.

After a contraction, there is a rest period for the heart. During these periods of repolarization, the heart goes through two stages: *absolute refractory,* when the heart cannot receive *any* stimulation, no matter how strong the impulse, and *relative refractory,* when the heart is susceptible to *strong* stimulation.

EXCUSE ME
When does the heart do all this?

Answer: Each and every time the heart beats, 60–100 times a minute. All day, all night, all year long.

All this electrical activity can be recorded on paper. That recording is known as an electrocardiogram, or ECG or EKG.

Conduction Pathways

Ode to a Node

Have a heart, and have no fear,
The SA node is over here.
Beating at a constant rate
60–100 is really great.
The AV node can make a show
if SA node has gone too slow.
40–60 is not too bad
If it's all you've got you will be glad.
Should the whole thing drop its speed
His and bundle branches will take the lead.
And that, my friend is the whole and part,
of the conduction system of your heart.

The electrical stimuli for the heart can be created by any myocardial cell, but usually it is created by primary pacemaker sites that are located throughout the heart. These sites are known as

- ❑ sinoatrial (SA) node (responsible for atrial contraction)
- ❑ atrioventricular (AV) node (the gatekeeper)
- ❑ bundle of His (named for its discoverer)[*]
- ❑ right and left bundle branches[*]
- ❑ Purkinje fibers[*]

SINOATRIAL NODE

The SA node is located in the upper right wall of the right atrium. The SA node is the primary pacemaker for the healthy heart for two reasons:

---

[*]Responsible for ventricular contraction.

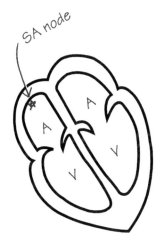

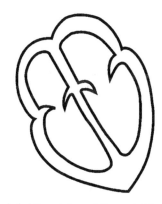

1. Label the atria and the ventricles.
2. Place a star at the SA node.

1. It is located *highest* in the heart, on the upper right wall of the atrium.
2. It has the *fastest* intrinsic firing rate: *60–100 beats per minute.* As long as the SA node continues to conduct impulses at this rate, no other pacemaker site feels the need to fire an impulse to pace the heart.

The intrinsic rate of the SA node is _____ beats per minute.

ANSWER: 60–100

EXCUSE ME
What do you mean by "intrinsic rate"?

Answer: "Intrinsic" means inborn, built in, or pre-set. The SA node is pre-set at the highest speed, 60–100 beats per minute. Other nodes of the heart, such as the AV node, monitor the heartbeat; if it drops below 50 beats per minute, they will take over pacing the heart.

The SA node fires impulses that contract the atria.

1. Place a star at the SA node.
2. Shade the atria.

SA node

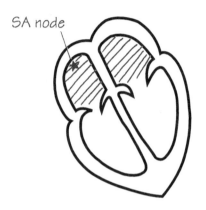

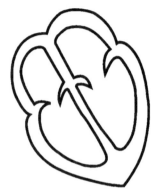

3. Fill in the intrinsic firing rate:
   _____ beats per minute.

4. The function of the SA node is to
   contract the _____.

Answers: 60–100; atria

ATRIOVENTRICULAR NODE

The AV node is located on the floor of the right atrium just above the ventricles.

Place a star on the AV node.

AV node

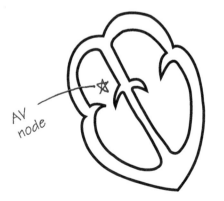

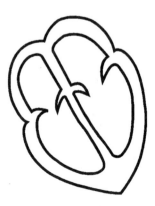

The function of the AV node is to act as a gatekeeper and briefly delay the impulses coming from the SA node, to allow the atria to contract completely and empty all of the blood into the ventricles.

If impulses are coming too fast, the AV node slows them. If impulses from the SA node are blocked or absent, the AV node can generate impulses to keep the heart beating.

Provided that the SA node does all it is supposed to do, the AV node just conducts impulses sent from above. The AV node has an intrinsic rate of *40–60 beats per minute*—slower than the SA node, but better than nothing.

Extra Credit

If the SA node were not firing and the AV node took over, what would be the heart rate (pulse) of the patient? It is a range of

_____ beats per minute.

ANSWER: 40–60

The AV node further conducts electrical impulses to the bundle of His. The bundle of His carries impulses from the AV node to the right and left bundle branches and eventually to the Purkinje fibers. These three systems together—the bundle of His, the left and right bundle branches, and the Purkinje fibers—are responsible for contracting the ventricles.

1. Divide the heart into the four chambers.
2. Star and label the SA node.
3. Star and label the AV node.
4. Draw and label the bundle of His.

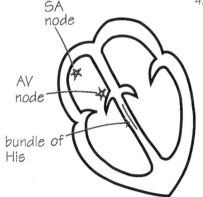

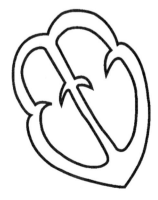

To contract fully, the ventricles require the assistance of the right and left bundle branches and the Purkinje fibers.

The excitation, or passage of an electrical impulse, along these pathways causes the ventricles to contract.

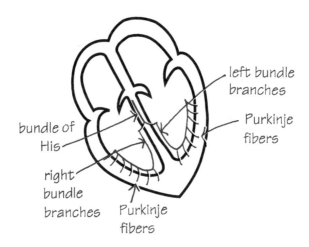

1. Outline the bundle of His, the right and left bundle branches, and the Purkinje fibers.
2. Shade the ventricles to show them contracting.

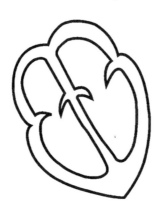

3. Fill in the intrinsic firing rate of the AV node: _____ beats per minute.
4. The function of the bundle of His, the left and right bundle branches, and the Purkinje fibers is to contract the _____.

Answers: 40–60; ventricles

The cells of the ventricles have the slowest intrinsic firing rate in the heart. They fire at 20–40 beats per minute.

The final phase of each heartbeat is the relaxation phase. In this relaxation or *refractory* phase, the heart relaxes and *repolarizes*.

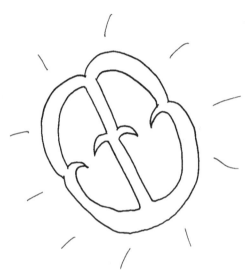

During the absolute refractory phase, the ventricles cannot receive further stimulation. As with other organs in the body, there is a period of time after stimulation when the ventricles cannot get excited again.

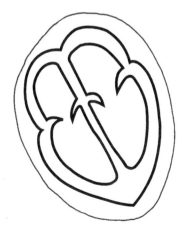

Circle the entire heart to show the heart relaxing and repolarizing.

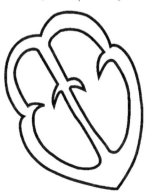

Let's review:

- ❏ *The SA node* is located in the upper right atrium. It has an intrinsic firing rate of 60–100 beats per minute and is the primary pacemaker for the heart.
- ❏ *The AV node* is located on the floor of the right atrium. It has an intrinsic firing rate of 40–60 beats per minute and is known as the gatekeeper of the heart because it regulates impulses coming from the SA node.
- ❏ *The bundle of His, the left and right bundle branches, and the Purkinje fibers* are located down the septum and in the lining of the ventricles. They have an intrinsic firing rate of 20–40 beats per minute. These three work together to contract the ventricles.

The ECG

Before Einthoven invented the electrocardiogram machine, patients had to be cut open to see what their heart was doing. This resulted in a generally poor prognosis. Now, we can monitor the heart's electrical activity through electrodes placed on intact skin.

The ECG records electrical conduction through the heart. Electrode pads placed on the patient's chest can detect the electrical activity generated by the myocardial cells. They are attached by cables to an ECG monitor. The ECG monitor has one positive electrode, one negative electrode, and one ground electrode.

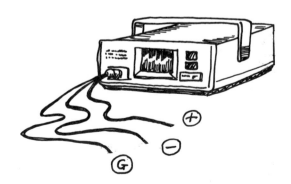

READING ECGs: P WAVES, QRS COMPLEXES, T WAVES

Atrial and ventricular depolarization and repolarization are electrical events that are seen as waves on an ECG monitor or on ECG paper. As the electrical impulse is conducted downward through the heart, we can watch its path on the ECG monitor. Each wave on the ECG represents the path of an electrical impulse as it is conducted through the heart.

P Wave

The P wave represents the depolarization (contraction) of the atria.

> 1. Place a star on the SA node.
> 2. Shade the atria.

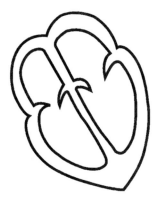

> 3. The function of the SA node is to contract the _____.
>
>   **Answer:** atria

A P wave.   Draw and label a P wave.

P-R Interval

The P-R interval is the time it takes for an electrical impulse to be conducted through the *atria and the AV node*. The P-R interval is measured from the *beginning* of the P wave to a small tail that extends just past the P wave. It is called the P-R interval, but it includes the entire P wave. It represents depolarization of the heart from the atria through the AV node. A normal P-R interval indicates that conduction through the AV node has followed a regular, unobstructed course.

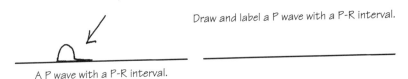

Draw and label a P wave with a P-R interval.

A P wave with a P-R interval.

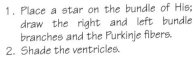

QRS Complex

The QRS complex represents the depolarization (contraction) of the ventricles.

1. Place a star on the bundle of His; draw the right and left bundle branches and the Purkinje fibers.
2. Shade the ventricles.

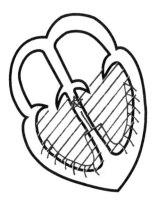

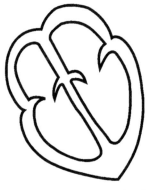

3. The function of the bundle of His, the right and left bundle branches, and the Purkinje fibers is to contract the _____.

Answer: ventricles

The QRS complex consists of

❑ The **Q** wave, which is the first negative or downward deflection of the complex. *The Q wave is often not seen.*

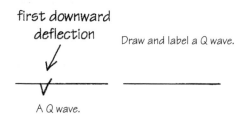

first downward
deflection

Draw and label a Q wave.

A Q wave.

❑ The **R** wave, which is the first upward deflection.

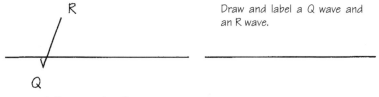

R

Draw and label a Q wave and an R wave.

Q

A Q wave and an R wave.

❑ *The S wave,* which is the rest of the complex, the next downward and upward deflection.

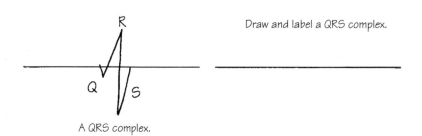

R

Draw and label a QRS complex.

Q   S

A QRS complex.

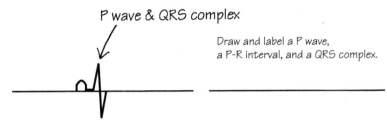

P wave & QRS complex

Draw and label a P wave,
a P-R interval, and a QRS complex.

A P wave, a P-R interval, and a QRS complex.

T Wave

The T wave represents the heart repolarizing (relaxing). This is called the refractory period.

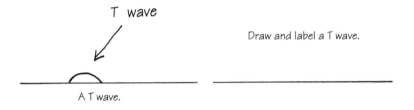

T wave

Draw and label a T wave.

A T wave.

The T wave is rounded. It is usually larger and more equally rounded than a P wave. Think of the shape of a turtle shell.

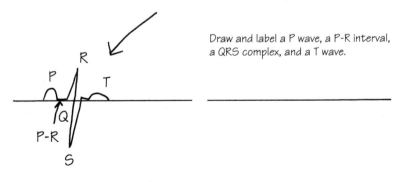

Draw and label a P wave, a P-R interval,
a QRS complex, and a T wave.

A P wave, a P-R interval, a QRS complex, and a T wave.

What would you see if the SA node didn't fire? Draw and label answer.

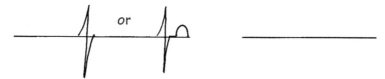

Answer: No P wave; QRS or QRS T only

What would you see if the SA node fired but the impulse was blocked at the AV node? Draw and label answer.

Answer: P wave only

What would you see if there was a delay at the AV node? Draw and label answer.

Answer: Long P-R interval

A Helpful Hint

Every patient's P waves, QRS complexes, and T waves look slightly different. If you are ever stuck and cannot distinguish which are the P waves and which are the T waves, try this: Find the QRS complex, and look *before* it: that should be a P wave. Look *after* it: that should be a T wave. Find another complex and try it again to check your first finding. This method works for most basic rhythms. To determine if a rhythm is regular, check the R-R interval. The R-R interval is measured from the peak of one R wave to the peak of the next (top of the QRS complex to top of the next QRS complex).

ECTOPIC ACTIVITY

All the cells in the heart can create electrical activity on their own. Usually, there is no need for this aberrant behavior, and cells quietly conduct impulses from the primary pacemaker sites. Occasionally, a little oxygen-deprived, irritable, frustrated cell goes off and fires on its own. This is known as *ectopic* or *aberrant* activity. Ectopic means outside of the usual pacemaker sites.

When this happens, the ectopic beat is recorded on the ECG as a different-looking complex. An oxygen-deprived, irritable cell is known as an *irritable focus,* or the plural, *irritable foci.*

If the ectopic beat is originating in an irritable focus close to the SA node, the beat looks almost like a normal P wave and conducts a normal looking QRS complex. There are two clues to recognizing an ectopic beat:

1. It looks slightly different.
2. It comes at an unexpected time.

Draw a complete complex.

_____

A complete complex.

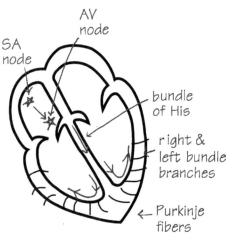

A regular path of conduction.

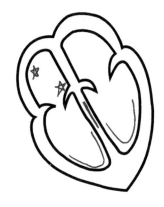

Outline the path of conduction.

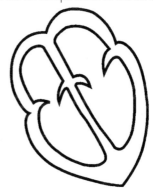

Draw an ectopic focus in the atria.

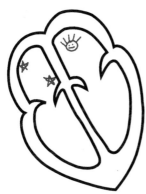

An ectopic focus in the atria.

Outline the path of conduction for this ectopic beat.

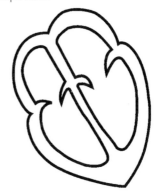

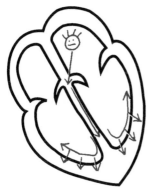

The path of conduction for this ectopic beat.

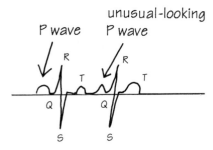

unusual-looking
P wave
P wave

Draw a complete complex followed by an unusual-looking P wave, a QRS complex, and a T wave.

A complete complex followed by an unusual-looking P wave, a QRS complex, and a T wave.

Premature Atrial Contraction

The beat just depicted is called a *premature atrial contraction:*

Premature meaning early or before the SA node was expected to fire.

Atrial meaning from the atria.

Contraction meaning beating or contracting of the heart.

It is from the atria because the impulse originated in the atria and it created a complex that looked like a P wave but not exactly like the other P waves, and it conducted a normal-looking QRS complex.

Two interesting facts to note:

1. The closer the irritable focus is to the SA node, the more the premature atrial contraction will resemble a P wave.

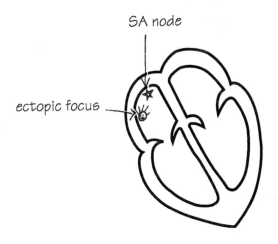

SA node

ectopic focus

2. The closer the irritable focus is to the AV node, the shorter the P-R interval.

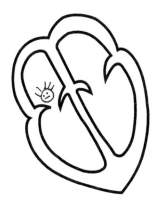

looks like
a P wave,
P wave   only a little different

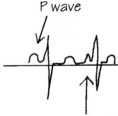

Close to the SA node, the premature atrial contraction looks like a P wave.

P wave

shortened P-R interval

Close to the AV node, the premature atrial contraction shortens the P-R interval.

EXCUSE ME
Why does the heart conduct these ectopic beats?

Answer: The cells of the heart conduct any electrical activity that reaches them regardless of origin. The heart cells have no way of knowing where the electrical activity originated. They conduct the beats in all directions, so if the atria are stimulated from below, they may conduct upward, resulting in a contraction from bottom to top.

Premature Junctional Contractions*

When the AV node fires on its own, there may be no P wave or there may be an inverted P wave (retrograde conduction).

---

*Also known as premature nodal contractions.

1. Draw the AV node firing.
2. Shade the ventricles.
3. Shade upward toward the bottom of the atrium.

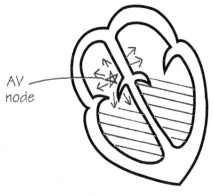

AV node

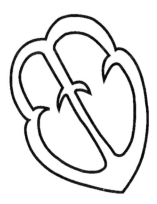

1. The AV node firing independently.
2. The shaded area contracts.

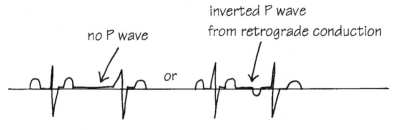

no P wave

inverted P wave
from retrograde conduction

or

A normal complex followed by a premature junctional contraction.
Draw a normal complex followed by a premature junctional contraction.

If the AV node becomes irritable or fussy and sends out a spark on its own, it results in

1. An inverted P wave or no P wave.
2. A stand-alone QRS complex and T wave.

This is called *nodal* or *junctional* because it originates in the AV node, also known as the AV junction.

If the impulse is conducted backwards up through the atrium, it may appear as an inverted P wave on the ECG.

Premature Ventricular Contractions

When an irritable or ectopic focus in the ventricle fires independently, it is called a premature ventricular contraction.

1. Draw an irritable focus in the ventricles.
2. Shade the ventricles to show them contracting.

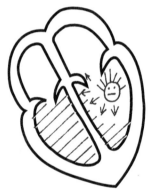 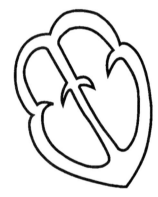

An irritable focus in the ventricles.

Because of the conduction pattern of a premature ventricular contraction, the complexes appear as wide and bizarre on the 3-lead ECG.

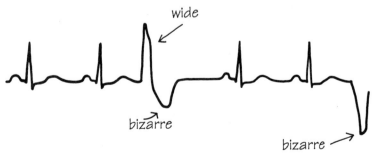

wide

bizarre

bizarre

A normal complex followed by a premature ventricular contraction.

Draw a normal complex followed by a premature ventricular contraction.

_____

There can be more than one ectopic focus in the ventricles. If so, the premature ventricular contractions look different from each other.

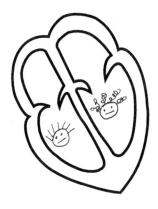

EXCUSE ME
How do I know if complexes are wide or thin or long or short? What does a normal complex look like?

Answer: Stay tuned.

Introduction to the Rhythms

ATRIAL FLUTTER

In atrial flutter, a single strong ectopic focus in the atrium starts to beat fast, 240–360 beats per minute. The AV node acts as a gatekeeper in this rhythm, allowing only some impulses through to the ventricles.

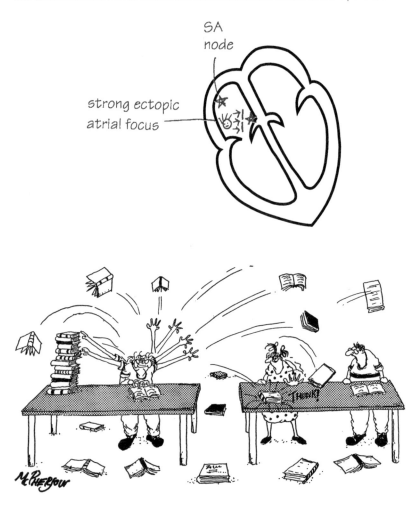

"He's been getting on my nerves ever since he took that speed reading course."

In atrial flutter, a single strong ectopic focus is sending out rapid impulses. (From CLOSE TO HOME Copyright John McPherson/Dist. of UNIVERSAL PRESS SYNDICATE. Reprinted with permission. All rights reserved.)

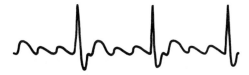

ATRIAL FIBRILLATION

In atrial fibrillation, many weak ectopic foci in the atria beat in an uncoordinated pattern, resulting in an uneven baseline of many tiny P waves known as fibrillatory (f) waves. Eventually the ventricles receive enough electrical stimulation to contract, or they contract on their own. This rhythm is characterized by a coarse baseline and an irregular distance between the QRS complexes.

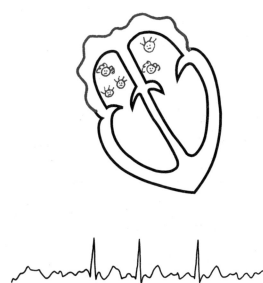

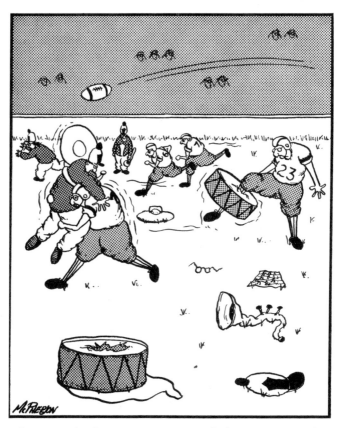

Apparently there was some confusion as to exactly when during the game the Fegley High Marching Band was supposed to perform.

In atrial fibrillation, many weak ectopic foci in the atria all fire at different times, causing an uncoordinated effort and confusion. (From CLOSE TO HOME Copyright John McPherson/Dist. of UNIVERSAL PRESS SYNDICATE. Reprinted with permission. All rights reserved.)

SUPRAVENTRICULAR TACHYCARDIA

This rhythm occurs when there is a fast, strong stimulus from an ectopic focus above the ventricles and below the SA node, and the heart conducts every beat. In supraventricular tachycardia the heart rate is 160–250 beats per minute.

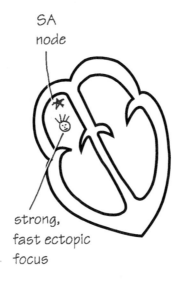

SA
node

strong,
fast ectopic
focus

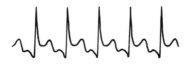

This can result in an inadequate refilling time, similar to squeezing a sponge fast under water and never allowing it to open or fill completely. This rapid action can result in low blood pressure. Additionally a person's heart cannot sustain this rhythm for long because the muscle itself gets tired.

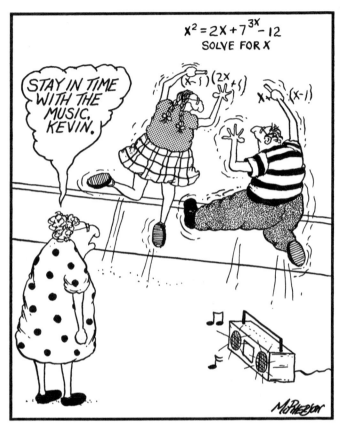

In an attempt to combine sports and academics, officials at Culver High devised aerobic algebra.

In supraventricular tachycardia, the impulses are conducted very fast, but it is almost impossible to sustain this rhythm. (From CLOSE TO HOME Copyright John McPherson/Dist. of UNIVERSAL PRESS SYNDICATE. Reprinted with permission. All rights reserved.)

VENTRICULAR TACHYCARDIA

Ventricular tachycardia is the result of one strong ventricular ectopic focus that hijacks the conduction system of the heart. This rhythm cannot sustain life for long. Ventricular tachycardia can be "stable," meaning with a pulse, or "unstable," meaning the patient is hemodynamically compromised, or pulseless.

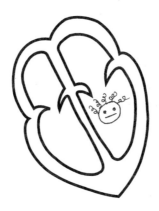

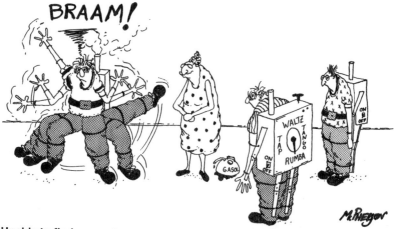

Unable to find guys who could dance in the school musical, choreographer Nelda Crantz develops and tests her automatic dancing machine.

Ventricular tachycardia has one strong ventricular focus. (From CLOSE TO HOME Copyright John McPherson/Dist. of UNIVERSAL PRESS SYNDICATE. Reprinted with permission. All rights reserved.)

VENTRICULAR FIBRILLATION

Ventricular fibrillation is the result of many weak ectopic foci in the ventricles, resulting in an uncoordinated undulation instead of a coordinated contraction. It is a rhythm that cannot circulate blood and is not compatible with life. If you could see the ventricles, they would resemble a squirming bag of worms.

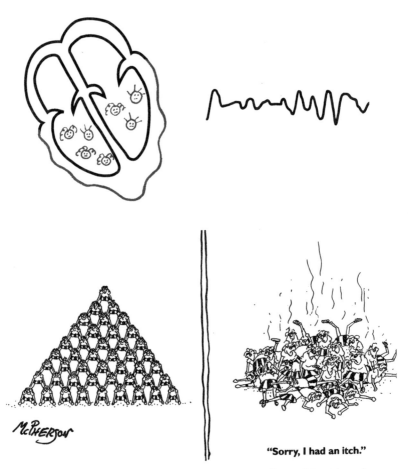

"Sorry, I had an itch."

Ventricular fibrillation is the result of the uncoordinated beating of many weak ectopic ventricular foci. (From CLOSE TO HOME Copyright John McPherson/Dist. of UNIVERSAL PRESS SYNDICATE. Reprinted with permission. All rights reserved.)

ASYSTOLE

Asystole, or a flatline, is not a rhythm but the absence of all electrical activity and is indicative of clinical death.

HEART BLOCKS

Heart blocks most commonly affect the AV junction. The impulse is either slowed at the AV junction or stopped at the AV junction.

Place a block at the AV junction.

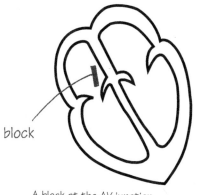

block

A block at the AV junction.

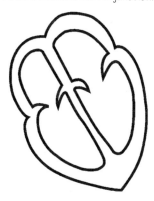

There are four types of AV blocks.

First Degree AV Heart Block

In first degree AV heart block the impulse is delayed at the AV junction. This results in a prolonged P-R interval.

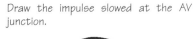

Draw the impulse slowed at the AV junction.

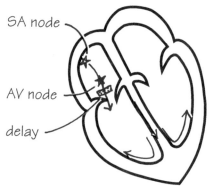

SA node

AV node

delay

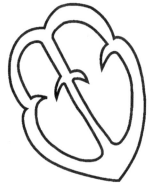

The impulse is slowed at the AV junction.

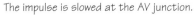

Draw a P wave with a prolonged P-R interval.

prolonged
P-R interval

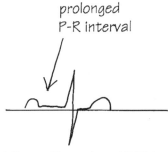

A P wave with a prolonged P-R interval.

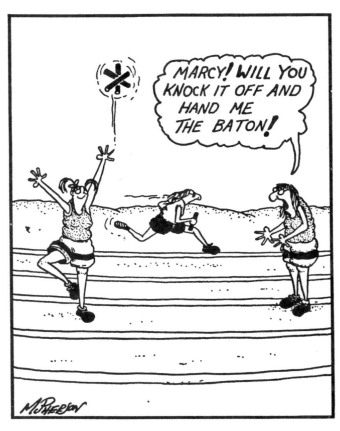

Majorettes make lousy relay racers.

In first degree AV heart block there is a delay at the AV node. (From CLOSE TO HOME Copyright John McPherson/Dist. of UNIVERSAL PRESS SYNDICATE. Reprinted with permission. All rights reserved.)

Second Degree AV Heart Block, Mobitz
Type I (Wenckebach)

Second degree AV heart block, Mobitz type I is characterized by a progressively increasing, abnormally long delay at the AV node causing a longer and longer P-R interval until no complex is conducted.

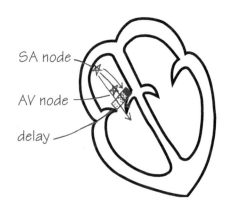

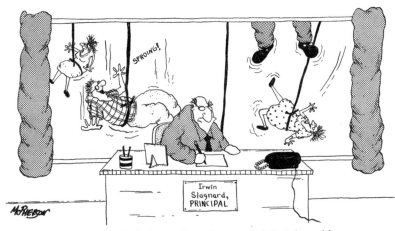

The third period chem. class discovered that the rubber tubing used in the lab is great for bungee jumping.

In Wenckebach, the delay gets longer and longer until it skips a beat. (From CLOSE TO HOME Copyright John McPherson/Dist. of UNIVERSAL PRESS SYNDICATE. Reprinted with permission. All rights reserved.)

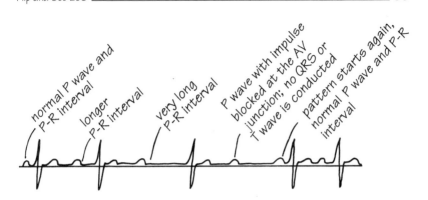

Second Degree AV Heart Block, Mobitz Type II

This heart block is characterized by an intermittent block at the AV node that conducts some impulses normally but completely blocks others. In this illustration, every other impulse is conducted.

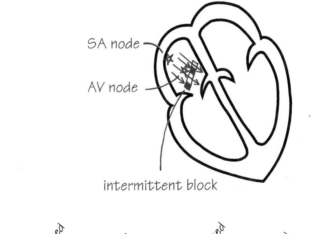

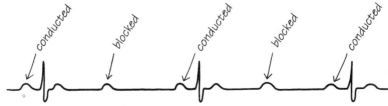

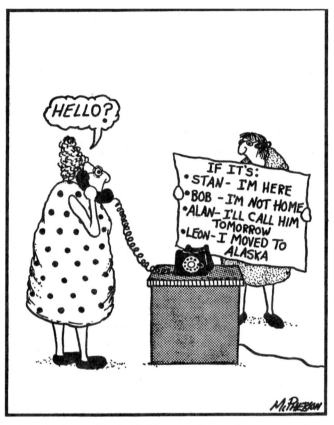

In second degree heart block, Mobitz type II impulses are conducted in a ratio. (From CLOSE TO HOME Copyright John McPherson/Dist. of UNIVERSAL PRESS SYNDICATE. Reprinted with permission. All rights reserved.)

Complete Heart Block

In third degree, or complete, heart block there is no communication between the atria and the ventricles. The P waves are generated by the atria, and the QRS complexes are being generated by the ventricles independently.

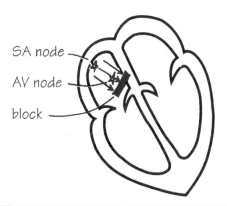

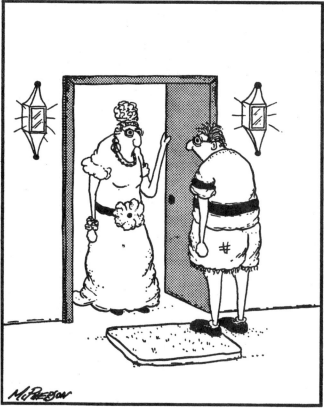

**Obviously there was some misunderstanding about
where Ray and Wanda were going on their date.**

In third degree heart block, there is no communication between the atria and the ventricles. (From CLOSE TO HOME Copyright John McPherson/Dist. of UNIVERSAL PRESS SYNDICATE. Reprinted with permission. All rights reserved.)

independent ventricular QRS complexes

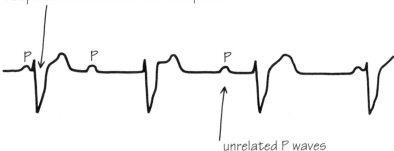

unrelated P waves

ARTIFICIAL PACEMAKERS

Pacemakers are battery-operated electrical devices that can fire either "on demand," meaning when the heart rate drops below a certain speed, or at a pre-set rate. They can be located anywhere in the heart but are usually placed in the ventricles.

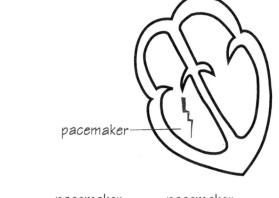

pacemaker

normal complex

pacemaker spike

pacemaker spike

wide QRS

wide QRS

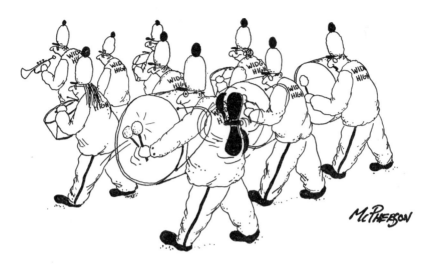

I'm tellin' ya, there's something weird about that new guy."

Electrical pacemakers are placed in the heart to keep the rate and rhythm regular and to keep it from dropping below a set speed. (From CLOSE TO HOME Copyright John McPherson/Dist. of UNIVERSAL PRESS SYNDICATE. Reprinted with permission. All rights reserved.)

ECG Paper

The complexes measure the events; the paper measures time. The ECG paper rolls out of the machine at a pre-set speed of 25 mm or 1 inch per second. The paper is marked off in a grid, with each line 1 mm apart. Every fifth line is darker and thicker. This is designed to help you count these very small boxes.

The small boxes represent 0.04 second. Each large box is made of five small boxes and represents 0.20 second.

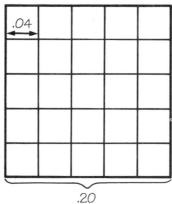

An event that takes 0.08 second would create a line two small boxes long.

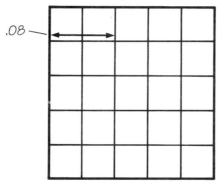

Draw a line representing 0.08 second (or two small boxes).

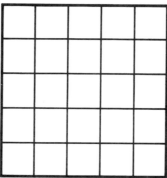

Draw a line representing 0.20 second (or one large box).

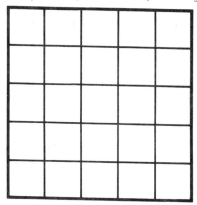

Draw a line representing 0.12 second. (How many boxes?)

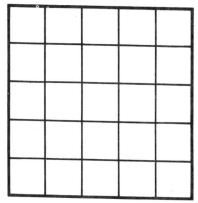

ANSWER: three small boxes long

Normal ECG

What is normal?

The criteria for a normal ECG are reproduced on the back of *Cohn's Pocket Guide to ECG Interpretation* and are as follows:

   one small box—0.04 second

   one large box—0.20 second

   P wave—3 small boxes or 0.12 second wide

   P-R interval—(count from the beginning of the P wave to the beginning of the R wave) 3–5 small boxes or 0.12–0.20 second wide

QRS complex—1–2½ small boxes or 0.04–0.10 second wide
   The height of the QRS is adjustable on each machine.

T wave—upright, well rounded, and less than half the height
   of the QRS complex

If it usually takes you 20 minutes to get to work and you are delayed in traffic, it will take you longer. You will use more gas and more time, even though you have traveled the same distance. Someone tracking you on radar would see a dot moving slowly across the screen.

In ECGs, if the *complex* is wider than normal, it means that the electrical impulse was slowed somewhere in the heart. If the complex is narrower than normal, it means that the impulses are passing more quickly through the heart.

The ECG is a graphic representation of the *electrical* activity in the heart. By counting the boxes, we can establish the time the complex took to travel. By counting the number of complexes in 1 minute, we can establish a rate.

Calculating Rate

It is unwieldy and cumbersome to count 60 seconds of ECG strip. There are a number of methods that have been established to count rate. Rulers are also available to assist in this calculation.

The easiest, most accurate method is called the *6-second strip method*. Instead of counting the number of complexes in *60* seconds, we count the number of complexes in *6* seconds and multiply by *10* (or just add a zero).

Six seconds of strip is equal to

❑ thirty large boxes (6 seconds) or

❑ six 1-second markers (6 seconds) or

❑ two 3-second markers (6 seconds) or

❑ one 6-second marker (6 seconds)

depending on design of the ECG strip you are using.

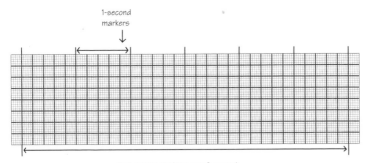

six 1-second markers, one 6-second
marker, or 30 large boxes

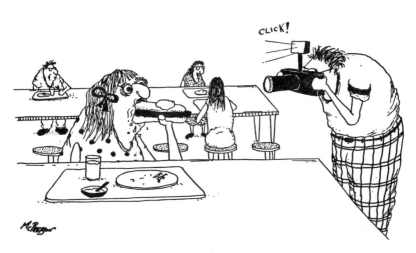

Timing is an essential part of being a yearbook photographer.

In ECG interpretation, timing is everything. (From CLOSE TO HOME
Copyright John McPherson/Dist. of UNIVERSAL PRESS SYNDICATE.
Reprinted with permission. All rights reserved.)

Practice calculating rate.

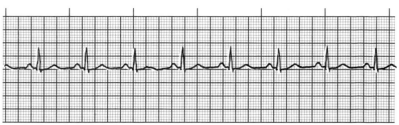

Rate is _____ beats per minute.

Answer: 80

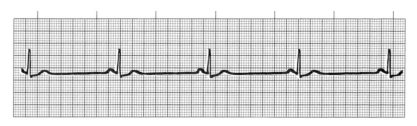

Rate is _____ beats per minute.

Answer: 40

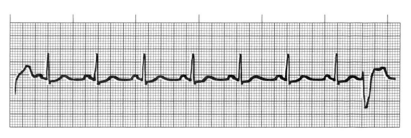

Rate is _____ beats per minute.

Answer: 70

Hint: Do not count the premature ventricular contraction.

Summary

Contraction and relaxation of the heart are mechanical events launched by electrical activity. The ECG is usually a good reflection of the current status of the heart. But not always.

You must confirm that what you see on the monitor is what is happening inside the patient; you should feel a pulse each time you see a complex on the monitor and should perform frequent blood pressure checks. In all cases, *you should always treat the patient and not the monitor.*

The ECG records the *electrical activity* of

1. The atria as they depolarize (the P wave).

2. The ventricles as they depolarize (the QRS complex).

3. The relaxation phase of the ventricles (the T wave); when the entire heart rests, relaxes, and repolarizes.

In most cases, the electrical activity of the heart accurately reflects the mechanical action inside.

The ECG records any and all electrical impulses in the heart. It records complexes that originate from primary pacemaker sites: the SA node, the AV node, the bundle of His, the left and right bundle branches, and the Purkinje fibers. It also records untoward, unwelcome impulses from elsewhere. The primary pacemaker sites usually lead to a regular rhythm, in which the R-R interval (the measure from R wave peak to R wave peak) remains constant.

Because all the cells of the heart can create their own electrical impulses, a phenomenon known as *automaticity,* we occasionally see *ectopic* pacemaker sites. Ectopic means outside or away from the usual pacemaker sites, as an ectopic pregnancy is one that is outside the uterus.

Complexes that look the same come from the same place in the heart. That place can be either a primary pacemaker such as the SA node or an ectopic pacemaker such as one small irritable, oxygen-deprived cell in the atria.

If the heart is ready to receive an electrical stimulation, it conducts any impulse that comes along and the ECG monitor or paper records it.

Naming Rhythms

To have success in naming rhythms, you'll need the following vocabulary:

sinus—normal
brady-—slow
tachy-—fast
-cardia—pertaining to the heart
regular—the R-R interval is equal
irregular—the R-R interval is irregular
premature—the complex came earlier than expected
compensatory—pause when the heart holds a beat
atrial—originating in the atria
ventricular—originating in the ventricles
contraction—an electrical impulse was conducted and contracted the heart muscle

ECGs are generally named for the pattern they represent.

It is like being a detective in a mystery game. All the clues are right here on the strips.

❑ Step 1—relax and get comfortable.

❑ Step 2—flip to the front of this book and pick up *Cohn's Pocket Guide to ECG Interpretation.*

❑ Step 3—read and answer the questions as they are listed on the pocket guide, and you'll be interpreting ECGs in the next 10 minutes.

Clues to Identifying Rhythms

The best approach to identifying rhythms is to use a systematic method, or a process that you repeat each time. One such system is presented by *Cohn's Pocket Guide to ECG Interpretation.* You should use that guide each time you identify a rhythm. Listed here are further pointers in ECG recognition.

1. Look for *complete complexes.* The QRS complex is the tallest complex. Find the QRS complex; *before* it is the P wave and

after it, the T wave. This doesn't always work, but it is always a good start.

2. Presence of *P* waves. Rhythms are usually named for their site of origin. Almost all rhythms with upright P waves originate in the atria.

3. *Rate* is the other clue to the origin of a rhythm. For example, a rate of 40–50 may be *junctional* because 40–50 beats per minute is the intrinsic firing rate of the AV junction. A rhythm strip with a rate of 44 and no P waves is junctional in origin.

4. Review the strip for *wildly abnormal beats*; calculate rate and name based on the underlying rhythm, not the abnormal beats. The presence of those beats may be the problem.

EXCUSE ME
What causes the heart to change rhythms?

Answer: Ectopic foci, damage to the heart muscle or the conduction pathway, or underlying medical conditions such as fever, hypoxia, and hypovolemia.

There are two basic kinds of rhythm disturbances:

1. *Rate* disturbances:
   ❏ too fast
   ❏ too slow
2. *Conduction* problems, including
   ❏ delays in conduction
   ❏ alternative pathways of conduction
   ❏ conduction of ectopic impulses
   ❏ metabolic imbalances

How to Use the Flip and See Portion of This Book

· ·

Please turn to the rhythm section of this book for the next exercise. To use the Flip and See rhythm section, you should

1. Separate the pages at the perforated line.
2. Flip just the right side of the book to create variations of rhythms.
3. Compare the rhythms side by side to see the differences in the patterns.

To use as a reference text, you can view rhythms in full strips across the page.

Flip and See Guided Tutorial

Here is a brief explanation of the defining characteristics of each rhythm. Try to view each rhythm as a pattern.

1. With both sides of *normal sinus rhythm* placed side by side, take a look at the pattern. All the intervals are regular and normal, with no bizarre ectopic activity. The rate is 80 beats per minute; the R-R intervals are regular. Count a 6-second strip.

2. *Flip just the right side of the page.* This is also a regular rhythm. If you check the R-R intervals, some are slightly uneven. This rhythm, *sinus arrhythmia,* results from the patient's normal breathing and is completely benign. The rate here is 70 beats per minute.

3. *Flip just the right side of the page.* All complexes are present, P-QRS-T, but this rhythm is slow: 40 beats per minute. The prefix *brady* means slow. This rhythm is *sinus brady-cardia.* It can be a normal finding in a well-trained athlete, but in an 87-year-old with an extensive cardiac history, it could be a sign of damage.

4. *Flip just the right side of the page.* This one looks normal but fast: 140 beats per minute. Anything over 100 is consid-

ered *sinus tachycardia. Tachy* means fast. This can be a response to certain conditions such as fever, fright, or hypoxia. When the rate starts to go very fast, P waves can be buried in the preceding complex.

5. *Flip just the right side of the page.* Just what are those peaks? Counting in from the left on the right-hand page and including the normal sinus beats, look at the first and sixth P waves. They are unusually shaped and come earlier than expected. They must be atrial in origin because the QRS complexes and T waves that follow are conducted normally. They are early atrial beats known as *premature atrial contractions.*

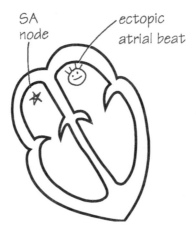

6. *Flip just the right side of the page.* Complex five (again, counting from the left on the right-hand page and including the normal sinus beats) is certainly wide and definitely bizarre looking. The wide ones appear different from each other, so they must be originating from different sites in the ventricles. These are called *multifocal premature ventricular contractions.* If all of the wide, bizarre complexes look the same, they are called *unifocal premature ventricular contractions* because they come from the same place in the ventricles.

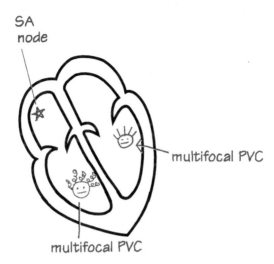

Multifocal foci create PVCs that look different from each other.

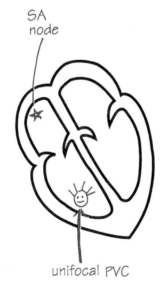

One single focus creates identical PVCs on a rhythm strip.

7. *Flip just the right side of the page.* Are there any P waves present, or are those all P waves? Actually, they are all *flutter* waves, also known as *F waves.* In *atrial flutter,* an ectopic focus in the atrium is beating fast, up to 350 beats a minute. In this case, the atria are beating at 210 times a minute. The AV node is acting as a gatekeeper and allowing only every third impulse to contract the ventricles. Only the QRS complex has the ability to create a pulse.

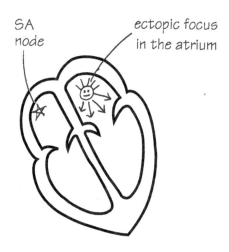

SA
node

ectopic focus
in the atrium

8. *Flip just the right side of the page.* This rhythm shows many weak ectopic foci in the atria. This produces an uncoordinated beating of the atria and "bag of worms" effect. In *atrial fibrillation,* the baseline may appear to have a few actual P waves but is made up mostly of *f waves.* The lower case "f" stands for fibrillatory waves. The R-R interval is irregular in this rhythm because occasionally one of these atrial impulses is strong enough to be conducted.

SA
node

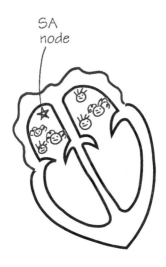

EXCUSE ME
How can you tell the difference between atrial fibrillation and normal sinus rhythm in a bouncy ambulance, where the baseline is wavy?

Answer: Check the R-R interval. Normal sinus rhythm has regular R-R intervals, whereas atrial fibrillation has irregular R-R intervals. In normal sinus rhythm with a bouncy baseline or a loose lead, the impulses are being conducted regularly, whereas in atrial fibrillation, the weak foci in the atria, with their sporadic conduction pattern, give it an irregular appearance. Place page 107 (Normal Sinus Rhythm with loose leads) and page 85 (Atrial Fibrillation) together and see the difference.

9. *Return the booklet to* normal sinus rhythm *on the left. Turn just the right side of the page to resume the lesson, on page 87.* Supraventricular tachycardia *or* paroxysmal supraventricular tachycardia *is a fast heart rate, 140–250 beats per minute, that originates above (supra) the ventricles, but below the SA node. It is characterized by a rapid heart rate,*

one so fast that sometimes the P wave runs into the preced-ing complex.

EXCUSE ME
How can I distinguish a fast sinus tachycardia from supraventricular tachycardia or paroxysmal supraventricular tachycardia?

Answer: (1) Look at the P wave. Sinus tachycardia's pacemaker is the SA node. The pacemaker for paroxysmal supraventricular tachycardia and supraventricular tachycardia is anything above the ventricles, **excluding** the SA node. (This will be a hard determination to make if the P waves are buried in the preceding complex.) (2) Check the rate. Sinus tachycardia's rate is 100–160 beats per minute. The rate for supraventricular tachycardia and paroxysmal supraventricular tachycardia is 160–250 beats per minute.

10. *Flip just the right side of the page.* This rhythm is ex-tremely dangerous: *ventricular tachycardia.* This is an ec-topic focus in the ventricles gone wild. Immediate interven-tion is needed here. The patient may be stable and talking, or unstable, or even pulseless.

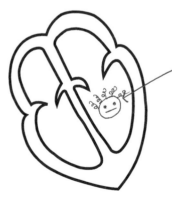

a very strong, dangerous ventricular ectopic focus

11. *Flip just the right side of the page.* This is *ventricular fibrillation*. The ventricles have become a "bag of worms." This rhythm does not move any blood and does not produce a heartbeat. This patient will present in cardiac arrest. Immediate defibrillation is what is needed here, in an attempt to get the heart back into a coordinated rhythm.

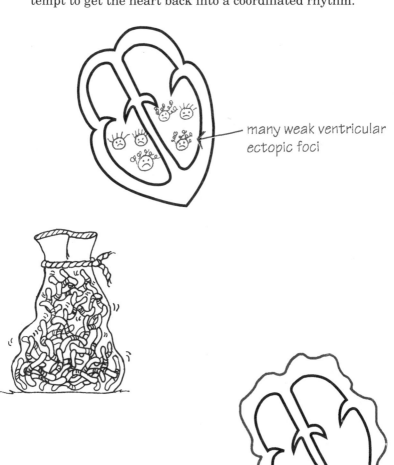

many weak ventricular ectopic foci

12. *Flip just the right side of the page.*
   - ❑ Clue #1—the rate is 40–60 beats per minute.
   - ❑ Clue #2—the P waves are inverted (retrograde) or missing.

This is a *junctional* or *nodal rhythm.* The rate produced by the junctional node is 40–60 beats per minute, and the conduction pattern is backward up through the atria and downward through the ventricles. We know there is retrograde conduction by looking at the upside-down P wave. If the P wave were absent, we would still call the rhythm *junctional* because it originated in the junction. There is also a rhythm known as *accelerated junctional,* which looks just like this one, with retrograde or absent P waves, but it is faster, above 60 beats per minute.

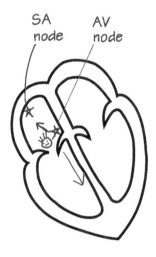

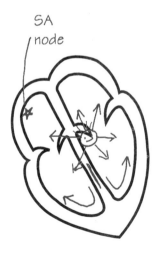

13. *Flip just the right side of the page.* This is not a rhythm. This is *asystole,* the absence of electrical activity in the heart, and is indicative of clinical death. *Remember always to check the patient's vital signs. The machine may not be "reading" the patient.*

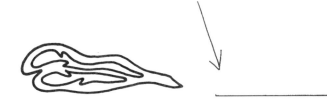

HEART BLOCKS

The next four rhythms represent delays or blockages in the electrical conduction system. See if you can determine where the blocks are occurring.

14. *Flip just the right side of the page.* Compare the normal sinus rhythm tracing on the left to the one on the right. What looks different? *The P-R interval is visually longer.* In this *first degree heart block,* there is a delay at the AV node, where the impulse becomes slowed. The normal P-R interval is 3–5 small boxes; the elongated one, 7–8 small boxes. At first glance, however, these rhythms look alike.
Do you think this is a dangerous rhythm?
No, it is not really dangerous by itself, but we might want to monitor the patient carefully to make sure that the impulses continue to get through. If they became blocked completely, instead of just delayed, it could become a serious condition.

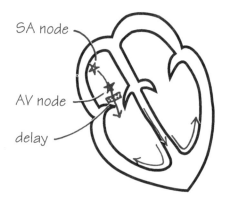

15. *Flip just the right side of the page.* This is another type of AV junction delay. Check your P-R intervals starting on the right-hand page at the first complex from the left. It gets longer and longer until it drops a QRS complex and a T wave. This rhythm is *second degree heart block, Mobitz type I, or Wenckebach,* characterized by a P-R interval that gets progressively longer until the impulse is blocked, and just a lone P wave appears.

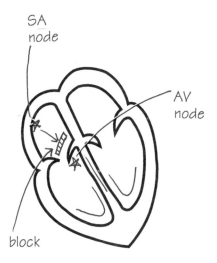

16. *Flip just the right side of the page.* In second degree heart block, Mobitz type II, some impulses are conducted normally while others are blocked. This can lead to a dangerous situation.

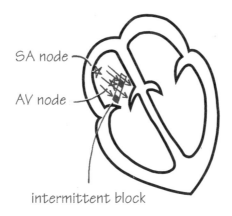

intermittent block

17. *Flip just the right side of the page.* This last actual rhythm is difficult to see and distinguish. It is called *complete heart block.* There is no relationship between the P waves and the QRS complexes. Every P wave is blocked.

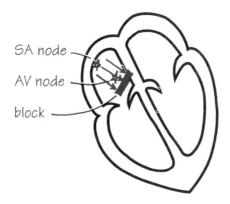

There are two clues. Impulses originating in the atria are at a normal rate of 60–100 and are regular. The ventricles, which are not receiving any stimulation from the atria (because the impulse is blocked at the AV node), are beating at a normal ventricular rate of 20–40 beats per minute and are regular. The ventricular beats look wide and unusual because they are originating in the ventricles. This is known as *third degree* or *complete heart block.*

18. *Flip just the right side of the page.* This rhythm is an *artificial pacemaker with capture.* The spikes preceding each complex are the pacemaker discharging and the electrical conduction system of the heart responding.

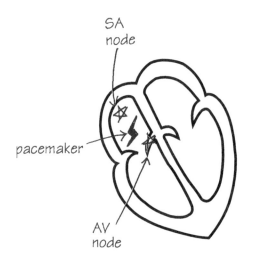

LOOK-ALIKE RHYTHMS

Place these rhythms next to each other for a demonstration of the differences:

1. Normal sinus rhythm and first degree heart block.
2. Second degree heart block, Mobitz type I, and second degree heart block, Mobitz type II.
3. Sinus tachycardia and supraventricular tachycardia.
4. Atrial flutter and atrial fibrillation.

NONRHYTHMS

19. *Flip just the right side of the page.* This rhythm has a wavy baseline but a regular R-R interval. You could compare it to atrial fibrillation by putting them side by side. This rhythm is actually a normal sinus rhythm with patient movement or a loose lead.

20. *Flip just the right side of the page.* This is a normal sinus rhythm with 60-cycle interference and is like static on the television set. Interference is generated inside the machine and can be resolved by moving away from the electrical current causing the interference.

PULSELESS ELECTRICAL ACTIVITY

EXCUSE ME

What about pulseless electrical activity?

Answer: Pulseless electrical activity (formerly known as electromechanical disassociation) is a condition in which you see a rhythm on the monitor, but the patient does not have a pulse. This can be caused by a variety of underlying medical emergencies that need to be addressed immediately. These conditions include

❑ Hypovolemia
❑ Hypoxia
❑ Cardiac tamponade
❑ Drug overdose
❑ Acidosis
❑ Tension pneumothorax
❑ Hypothermia
❑ Massive pulmonary embolism
❑ Hyperkalemia
❑ Massive acute myocardial infarction

The treatment for pulseless electrical activity is as follows:

1. Cardiopulmonary resuscitation (CPR) should be initiated on all pulseless patients regardless of the rhythm.

2. Advanced cardiac life support (ACLS) resuscitation should be initiated: intubation, intravenous access, medication.

3. Investigate and treat underlying cause.

Summary: This patient will have a visible electrical activity on the cardiac monitor but will not have a palpable pulse. This means that the heart's *electrical system* is functioning but that there is a problem with other connected systems. There may be a mechanical pump problem, a vascular system problem, metabolic imbalance, or a drug overdose. These underlying problems have to be addressed for the resuscitation to be successful.

Summary and a Few Golden Rules

ECG monitor interpretation is a visual skill that is developed by practice and feedback. It is like going to work in a new office and learning the names of your co-workers. In the beginning, it is hard; there may even be two people who look alike; often there is one person whose name you *always* forget. In a matter of days, you find that you can name one or two people; in weeks you can name more. Occasionally, you will get on the elevator with someone who works in the basement and you'll think "I've never seen *that* woman before." And so it is with ECG recognition, especially if you are in a place where there are a lot of people on cardiac monitors. Some rhythms will start to look like old friends (especially the normal ones, because you breathe a sigh of relief when you see them). Some will cause you great anxiety. This book is designed to cover only the most basic rhythms. As you continue your practice, you may, and likely will, see rhythms not included here. If you happen on an unusual or interesting rhythm, print a strip, label it, and slip it in this book. That way you'll create your own advanced version of this book.

EXCUSE ME
Are these rhythms from real people?

Answer: Most of these are real rhythms taken from patients in the Emergency Department. Some rhythms are computer generated. Here are two more real rhythms; the first is a junctional rhythm, and the second is a normal sinus rhythm (with a rate of 100 beats per minute). Some variation is present, but you can easily recognize these rhythms. Although some of the more unusual rhythms are not included in this book, and some of the regular rhythms have obscure presentations, you should now have enough knowledge to start. Good luck.

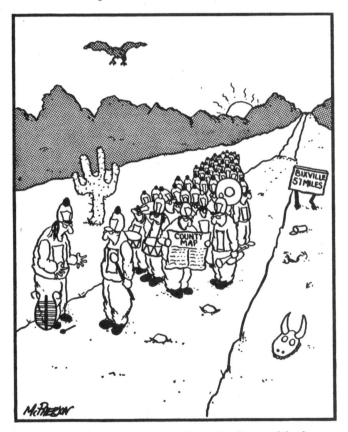

"All you had to do was follow the float with the pink cows! Was that so hard?!"

Arrhythmias can occur when electrical impulses are conducted in an unusual manner. (From CLOSE TO HOME Copyright John McPherson/Dist. of UNIVERSAL PRESS SYNDICATE. Reprinted with permission. All rights reserved.)

Golden Rules

1. Always treat the *patient,* not the monitor.
2. *Always* take a pulse and blood pressure.
3. Patients with an impending feeling of doom should be taken seriously.
4. *Don't panic.* If the patient is talking to you, then you probably have a minute to think of what to do next. While you are thinking, give the patient some oxygen.
5. Patients in complete cardiac arrest are actually easy to treat; just follow your ACLS protocols.
6. It is harder to read a screen than to read a strip. If you are uncertain of the rhythm, run a strip and see if that helps.
7. Use *Cohn's Pocket Guide to ECG Interpretation;* it may help you to remember the name of a rhythm, and it is always handy to have a small ruler.
8. When faced with an unusual presentation (e.g., the rhythm does not match the clinical presentation of the patient), check the patient, the leads, and the monitor.
9. Intravenous lines are easier to start while the person still has a blood pressure; try to get early intravenous access.
10. Ask for help if you need it. Request direction if you are unsure of what to do next.

Rhythms

NORMAL SINUS RHYTHM

NORMAL SINUS RHYTHM

Name: Normal sinus rhythm (regular sinus rhythm)

Description: 60–100 beats per minute
Each complex is complete: P wave, QRS complex, T wave
No untoward, wide, bizarre, ectopic, early, late, or different-looking complexes
All intervals within normal limits

Treatment: Monitor vital signs; check blood pressure

Questions: AMPLER

Next Step: Monitor patient's condition

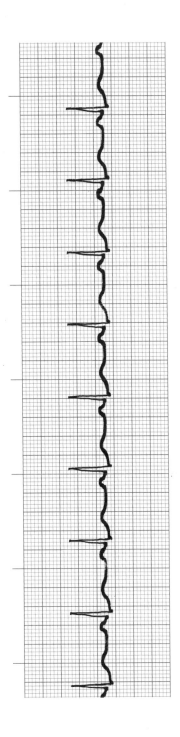

SINUS ARRHYTHMIA

Name: Sinus arrhythmia (normal variation)

Description: 60–100 beats per minute

Each complex is complete: P wave, QRS complex, T wave

No untoward, wide, bizarre, ectopic, early, late, or different-looking complexes

All intervals except R-R within normal limits

Treatment: Monitor vital signs

Questions: AMPLER

Next Step: Monitor patient's condition; sinus arrhythmia is a natural variation caused by normal breathing

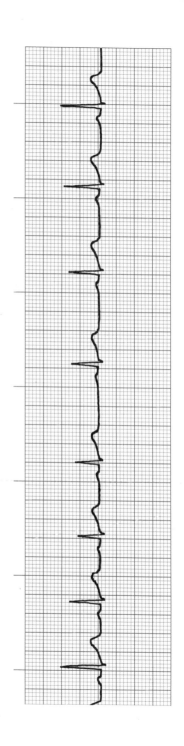

SINUS BRADYCARDIA

Name: Sinus bradycardia (normal slow)

Description: Less than 60 beats per minute
Each complex is complete: P wave, QRS complex, T wave
No untoward, wide, bizarre, ectopic, early, late, or different-looking complexes
All intervals *except rate* within normal limits

Treatment: Monitor vital signs; check blood pressure; may be normal in the young and healthy. If blood pressure is normal, no other treatment is required. If patient is hypotensive, "shocky," cool, or clammy or has chest pain or a change in mental status, consider **ATROPINE**. If ectopic activity is present, consider atropine before lidocaine

Continued on following page

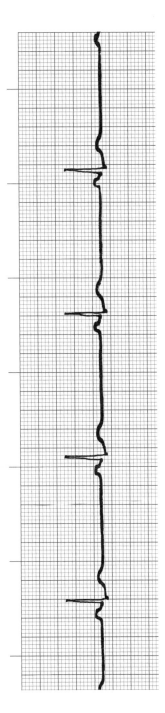

Questions: AMPLER. Do you take digitalis, propranolol, or quinidine?

Next Step: Consider acute myocardial infarction, digitalis toxicity, calcium channel blocker overdose, and electrical conduction system damage. Monitor blood pressure, check cardiac monitor for ectopic activity related to low rate, consider vasovagal response, treat underlying cause

SINUS TACHYCARDIA

Name: Sinus tachycardia (normal fast)

Description: 100–160 beats per minute

Each complex is complete: P wave, QRS complex, T wave.

Note: P waves may be buried in the previous T wave

No untoward, wide, bizarre, ectopic, early, late, or different-looking complexes

All intervals *except rate* are within normal limits

Treatment: Monitor vital signs; check blood pressure; treat the underlying condition

Questions: AMPLER. Do you take digoxin?

Continued on following page

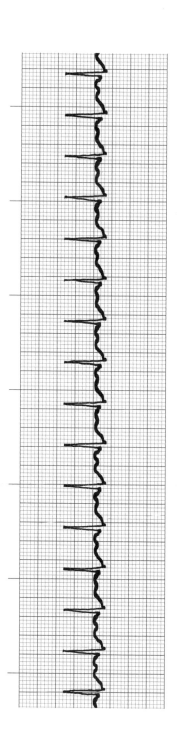

Next Step: Tachycardia can be caused by fear/anxiety, fever, hypoxia, shock, congestive heart failure, medications, pain, cocaine/crack, and blood loss. At very fast rates, the heart cannot refill fully, leading to reduced cardiac output. In the setting of ischemia, this hard work can further damage the heart muscle

PREMATURE ATRIAL CONTRACTIONS

PREMATURE ATRIAL CONTRACTIONS

Name: Premature atrial contractions (early ectopic atrial activity)

Description: Usually 60–100 beats per minute, but varies depending on the number of extra atrial beats that are created and conducted and on the rate of the underlying rhythm.

Premature atrial contractions are ectopic beats that occur in the context of other rhythms

Each complex is complete: P wave, QRS complex, T wave

The early P waves look different from the normal P waves. These early P waves may be smaller or peaked. The QRS complex may be normal or conducted differently

Continued on following page

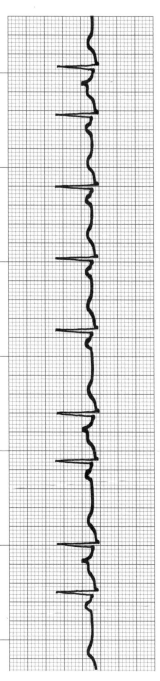

P-R intervals may vary (usually shorter) depending on the distance from the ectopic foci to the AV node

R-R interval varies at the ectopic complex

Treatment: Monitor vital signs; watch for change in rhythm

No other treatment is necessary

Questions: AMPLER

Next Step: Premature atrial contractions may be a normal finding

PREMATURE VENTRICULAR CONTRACTIONS

PREMATURE VENTRICULAR CONTRACTIONS

Name: Premature ventricular contractions (early ectopic ventricular complexes)

Description: Rate depends on underlying rhythm. Do *not* count the premature ventricular contraction

Premature ventricular contractions are ectopic beats that occur in the context of other rhythms. Premature ventricular contractions are not a rhythm themselves

The premature ventricular contraction is an untoward, wide, bizarre, early, and different-looking complex. If there is just one ectopic focus, the premature ventricular contraction is called unifocal and each one looks the same. If there is more than one ectopic focus, the premature ventricular contractions are called multifocal and vary in appearance

Continued on following page

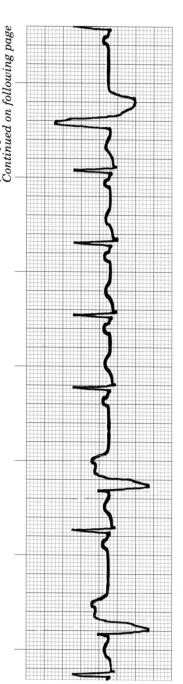

Intervals may be irregular owing to the premature complexes and compensatory pauses. No P waves are present before the premature ventricular contraction

Treatment: Monitor vital signs, check blood pressure. *Occasional premature ventricular contractions with no symptoms require no treatment.* Premature ventricular contractions in the presence of acute myocardial infarction/chest pain, frequent multifocal or unifocal premature ventricular contractions, greater than six per minute, or back-to-back premature ventricular contractions may require treatment with **LIDOCAINE**

Questions: AMPLER/PQRST

Next Step: Monitor patient's condition. Watch the monitor for runs of premature ventricular contractions or a change in rhythm

82

ATRIAL FLUTTER

ATRIAL FLUTTER

Name: Atrial flutter (F waves) (very rapid atrial rate; think of atrial *fluuuuuuuter*)

Description: Atrial flutter is a fast, constant, firing of an ectopic focus
The *atrial* rate is very fast, 240–360 beats per minute.
Instead of P waves, atrial flutter has F waves
The *ventricular* rate depends on the conduction ratio, 2:1, 3:1, 4:1, usually 60–100 beats per minute
The complexes are incomplete. They start with F waves as a baseline: *F wave, F wave, QRS complex, F wave (with T wave buried in the F wave) F wave*
Baseline consists of constant F waves and intermittently conducted QRS complexes, and if you turn the rhythm strip upside down it is thought to resemble a sawtooth pattern

Continued on following page

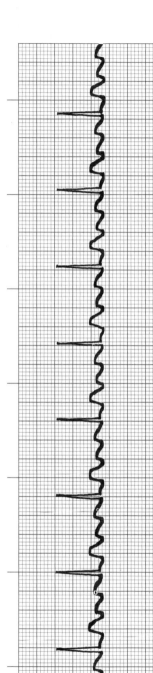

Intervals cannot be measured because there is no
P wave. QRS complexes are usually within normal
limits. T waves usually cannot be seen

Treatment: Hemodynamically stable patients (no signs of shock)
require no initial treatment
If *ventricular* (QRS) rate is rapid, 120–140 beats per
minute, consider cardioversion, digitalis,
or propranolol
Monitor vital signs; check blood pressure

Questions: AMPLER/PQRST
Do you take digitalis?

Next Step: Monitor patient's condition; frequent blood pressure
and rhythm checks

ATRIAL FIBRILLATION

Name: Atrial fibrillation (f waves) (uncoordinated, fast atrial activity)

Description: *Atrial* rate appears as the baseline 350–600 beats per minute. May be coarse (and able to be counted) or so fine they appear too small to count. There are no P waves; instead atrial fibrillation has **f** waves, known as fibrillatory waves

Ventricular rate is 100–160 beats per minute. R-R interval is always irregular because of chaotic constant stimulation from the atria

Baseline is all f waves, with QRS complexes usually within normal limits

Continued on following page

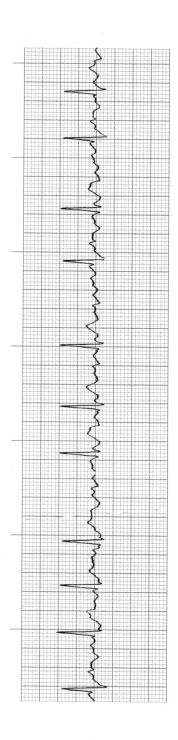

Treatment: In the hemodynamically stable patient, no treatment is required. This may be normal for elderly patients
In the unstable patient (syncope, signs/symptoms of shock), monitor vital signs and check blood pressure

. Consider cardioversion and digitalis.

Questions: AMPLER/PQRST. Do you have chest pain?
Do you take digoxin, verapamil, or propranolol?

Next Step: Atrial fibrillation can lead to reduced cardiac output up to 20% and a danger of clot formation from poor atrial emptying

SUPRAVENTRICULAR TACHYCARDIA

SUPRAVENTRICULAR TACHYCARDIA

Name: Supraventricular tachycardia (paroxysmal supraventricular tachycardia) (fast rate from a pacemaker site above the ventricles)

Description: 160–250 beats per minute

Each complex is complete: P wave, QRS complex, T wave, P waves may be absent or may be buried in the preceding complex

No untoward, wide, bizarre, ectopic, late, or different-looking beats except for P waves that may be absent or abnormal

QRS complex and T wave within normal limits. Rate is very fast

Continued on following page

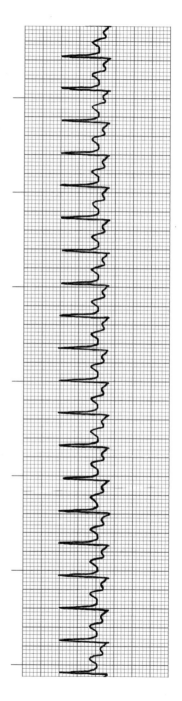

Treatment: Monitor vital signs; check blood pressure:
consider vagal maneuvers
consider drug intervention
consider cardioversion

Questions: AMPLER/PQRST. Listen to lung sounds

Next Step: Monitor patient for congestive heart failure,
signs/symptoms of shock

**VENTRICULAR
TACHYCARDIA**

VENTRICULAR TACHYCARDIA

Name: Ventricular tachycardia (rapid deadly rhythm of the ventricles)

Description: 100–250 beats per minute
Only wide, tall, bizarre-looking complexes
QRS complex greater than 0.12 second, wide, weird-looking

Treatment: **THIS IS A DEADLY RHYTHM.** The ventricles cannot maintain this rate
Monitor vital signs; check blood pressure
If patient is awake and alert with adequate vital signs, give lidocaine. Consider further drug therapy
If patient has no vital signs, treat as ventricular fibrillation with serial defibrillation and CPR
Continued on following page

Questions: **MONITOR ABCs. AMPLER.** How long has patient been like this?

Next Step: Monitor; intravenous access; defibrillation pads; CPR; prepare for cardiac arrest

VENTRICULAR FIBRILLATION

Name: Ventricular fibrillation (rapid, uncoordinated firing of the ventricles, like a "bag of worms")

Description: **THIS IS A DEADLY RHYTHM**
This rhythm does not generate a pulse
Completely uncoordinated electrical activity without any discernible complexes
All waves are **f** waves (fibrillatory waves)

Treatment: Quickly check vital signs. If none are present, defibrillate immediately
CPR/intravenous line/Advanced Cardiac Life Support protocol

Questions: How long has patient been like this? AMPLER

Next Step: Intubation; CPR; intravenous access

JUNCTIONAL (NODAL) RHYTHM

Name: Junctional (nodal) rhythm (originating in the AV junction)

Description: Usually 40–60 beats per minute, the intrinsic rate of the *AV node*

No preceding P waves because the impulse is generated in *AV node*. Occasionally P waves have retrograde conduction (deflected downward) either before or after the QRS complex

QRS complex and T wave usually normal

NOTE: Accelerated junctional rhythms meet the above criteria but are at a rate of 60–100 beats per minute

Treatment: Monitor vital signs. If vital signs and patient are stable, treat underlying cause: myocardial infarction, congestive heart failure, acidosis, hyperkalemia

Continued on following page

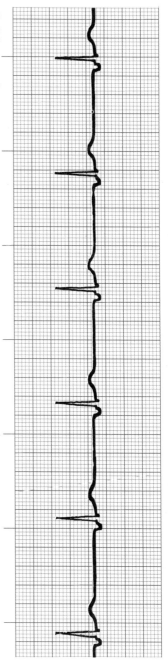

Establish intravenous access; prepare pacemaker

Questions: AMPLER/PQRST. Medications?

Next Step: Carefully monitor vital signs and mental status. Keep pacemaker and medications nearby

ASYSTOLE

ASYSTOLE

Name: Asystole (cardiac standstill/flat line)

Description: **THIS RHYTHM IS ASSOCIATED WITH DEATH**
No pulse
Less than 5 beats per minute
ECG shows underlying asystole with occasional agonal
beats
No complexes are associated with this rhythm

Treatment: Quickly check vital signs. CPR

Questions: How long has patient been like this? AMPLER

Next Step: Intubate, resuscitate, transport/transfer to ED/CCU, or
pronounce patient dead

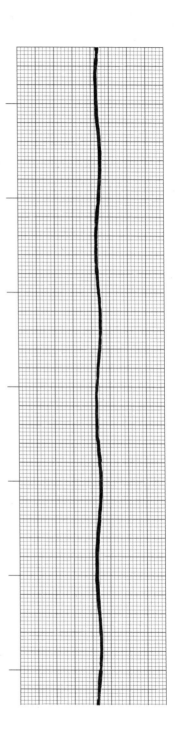

FIRST DEGREE AV HEART BLOCK

FIRST DEGREE AV HEART BLOCK

Name: First degree AV heart block (elongated P-R interval)

Description: 60–100 beats per minute

Each complex is complete: P wave, QRS complex, T wave

No untoward, wide, bizarre, ectopic, early, late, or different-looking beats

All intervals within normal limits, **EXCEPT** the **P-R interval** is greater than 0.20 second (or five small boxes)

Note: This rhythm looks just like normal sinus rhythm except that it has an elongated P-R interval. Flip to normal sinus rhythm to compare rhythms

Continued on following page

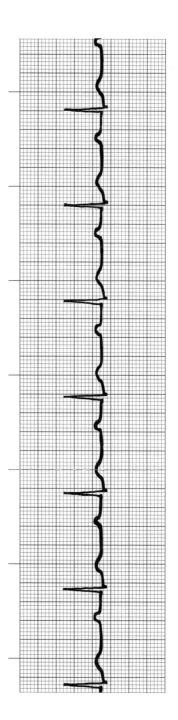

First degree AV heart block is a slowing at the AV node, creating a prolonged P-R interval. May be caused by damage to the junction, increased vagal tone, drug toxicity

Treatment: Monitor vital signs and check blood pressure. If patient is stable, no treatment is indicated

Questions: AMPLER/PQRST. Do you take digitalis or quinidine?

Next Step: Monitor patient's condition and watch for further deterioration of rhythm

SECOND DEGREE HEART BLOCK, MOBITZ TYPE I (WENCKEBACH)

Name: Second degree heart block, Mobitz type I (Wenckebach) (progressive lengthening of the P-R interval)

Description: 60–100 beats per minute

Almost every complex is complete: P wave, QRS complex, T wave, *except* some P waves are *not* followed by a QRS complex or a T wave because the impulse was blocked

No untoward, wide, bizarre, ectopic, early, or different-looking complexes

Continued on following page

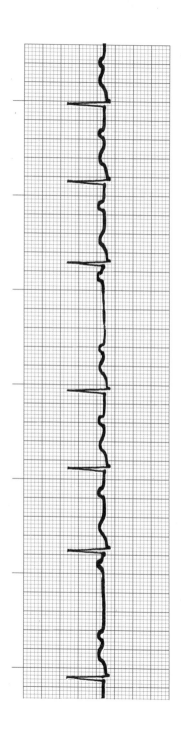

The P-R interval becomes longer and longer until the impulse is not conducted at all and the QRS complex and the T wave are missing. P--QRS-T, P---QRS-T, P------QRS-T, P--------- P--QRS--T. After the beat is dropped, the P-R interval returns to normal

All other intervals are within normal limits

Treatment: Monitor vital signs and blood pressure; if rate is below 60 beats per minute or vital signs are unstable, treat the bradycardia

Questions: AMPLER/PQRST

Next Step: Monitor patient's condition

SECOND DEGREE HEART BLOCK, MOBITZ TYPE II

SECOND DEGREE HEART BLOCK, MOBITZ TYPE II

Name: Second degree heart block, Mobitz type II (some impulses are conducted normally, and others are blocked)

Description: 30–100 beats per minute depending on the ratio of conduction: 2:1, 3:1, 4:1

Almost every complex is complete: P wave, QRS complex, T wave, *except* some P waves are *not* followed by a QRS complex or a T wave because the impulse is blocked

Impulses are blocked at the AV node so that some P waves stand alone

In type II heart block, the P-R interval is constant and normal

Continued on following page

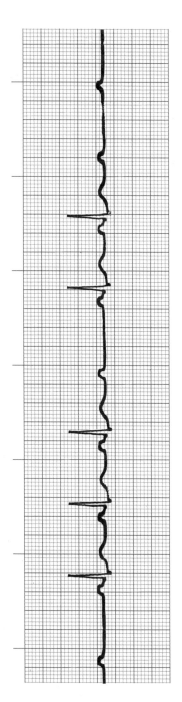

No untoward, wide, bizarre, ectopic, early, late, or different-looking complexes

All intervals *except* R-R are normal

Mobitz type II beats conduct in a ratio: 1:1, 2:1, 3:1, or 4:1

Treatment: Monitor vital signs; check blood pressure. If vital signs are stable; no treatment is indicated. Treatment is indicated if bradycardia persists or is symptomatic

Questions: AMPLER/PQRST

Next Step: Watch the patient and monitor for further deterioration

THIRD DEGREE AV HEART BLOCK: COMPLETE HEART BLOCK

THIRD DEGREE AV HEART BLOCK: COMPLETE HEART BLOCK

Name: Third degree AV heart block: complete heart block (no relationship between the P waves and QRS complexes)

Description: The AV node is completely blocked. There is no relationship between the P wave and the QRS complex/T wave P wave (atrial) rate 60–100 beats per minute QRS complex (ventricular rate 20–40 beats per minute). T waves follow QRS complexes QRS complexes may look narrow if the pacemaker is junctional, or wide and bizarre if the pacemaker is ventricular.

Continued on following page

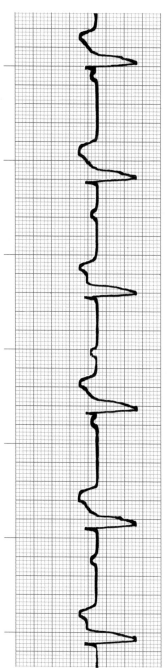

P-R interval varies because it is completely random and unrelated to QRS complex

Treatment: Monitor vital signs; check blood pressure; only *ventricular* beats produce a pulse. Blood pressure may be low. Cardiac output is compromised. If there are signs/symptoms of shock, give atropine. Do NOT give lidocaine

Consider a pacemaker

Questions: AMPLER/PQRST

Next Step: Carefully monitor patient until successfully medicated or paced

PACEMAKER WITH 1:1 CAPTURE

PACEMAKER WITH 1:1 CAPTURE

Name: Pacemaker rhythm (cardiac pacemakers deliver an electrical stimulus to the heart, causing electronic depolarization and subsequent cardiac contraction)

Description: Pacemakers can be transcutaneous (through the skin), transvenous (tip of the venous catheter in the right ventricle, right atrium, or both), transthoracic (through the anterior chest wall into the heart), epicardial (on the surface of the heart), or "permanent" (surgically implanted inside the heart). Depending on the type, pacemakers can be used externally in an emergency situation to keep the heart beating while an operating room is being prepared, or they can be surgically implanted.

Continued on following page

Occasionally they are used with severe tachycardia; this is called *overdrive* pacing. They can act as the primary pacemaker, or they can be set to activate if the heart rate drops below a pre-set number (demand)

On ECG they appear as straight, hard, vertical lines known as *pacemaker spikes*, each followed by a wide QRS complex and T wave (which may or may not look normal)

P waves may be absent or present, and they may or may not be associated with the QRS complexes. Functioning pacemakers produce spikes followed by QRS complexes

Capture (an electrical event) is achieved when each pacemaker spike is followed by a wide QRS complex and T wave. Patients in whom this occurs should always be assessed by taking a pulse and blood pressure

Treatment: Monitor vital signs; check pulse and blood pressure frequently. Notify cardiology of the need for a permanent pacemaker. Treat underlying rhythm, i.e., bradycardia, tachycardia, or complete heart block

Questions: AMPLER/PQRST. Do you have a pacemaker? Where is it located? How long have you had this pacemaker?

Next Step: Carefully monitor patient until successfully stabilized

LOOSE LEAD/CABLE MOVEMENT

LOOSE LEAD/CABLE MOVEMENT

Name: Loose lead/cable movement (artifact produced by extra movement of one or more of the electrodes)

Description: Improperly applied electrodes; loose, disconnected, or reversed leads or cables; inadequate electrode paste; oily skin; chest hair; excessive sweating or shivering; patient movement; muscle tremor; heavy or rapid breathing; a bumpy ambulance ride; use of other electric equipment around the monitor; and a variety of other factors can produce artifacts in the ECG, some of which bear an alarming resemblance to life-threatening dysrhythmias. An artifact can appear on a strip with any underlying rhythm. P waves, QRS

Continued on following page

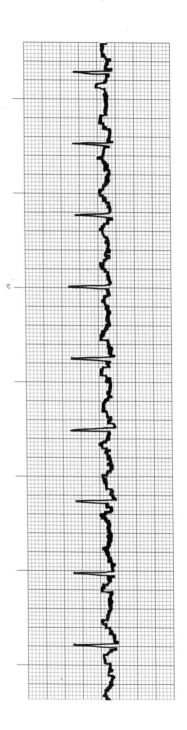

complexes, and T waves are dependent on the underlying rhythm

Treatment: Check pulse and blood pressure. Check the electrodes and cables for disconnection, placement over a bony prominence, chest hair, diaphoresis, inadequate contact, and placement. If patient is diaphoretic, use diaphoretic leads; if pediatric patient, use pediatric leads appropriate to patient's size

Next Step: Change cables, monitor, or leads, as appropriate

60-CYCLE INTERFERENCE

60-CYCLE INTERFERENCE

Name: 60-cycle interference

Description: This artifact is produced by electrical interference caused by a source of alternating current. 60-cycle is AC interference. The P waves, QRS complexes, and T waves reflect the underlying rhythm

Treatment: Move the cables away from the source of the interference

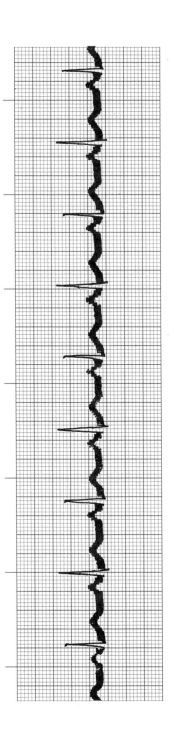

JUNCTIONAL RHYTHM WITH RATE OF 40 BEATS PER MINUTE

JUNCTIONAL RHYTHM WITH RATE OF 40 BEATS PER MINUTE

Name: Junctional (nodal) rhythm (originating in the AV junction)

Description: Usually 40–60 beats per minute, the intrinsic rate of the *AV node*
No preceding P waves because the impulse is generated in *AV node.* Occasionally P waves have retrograde conduction (deflected downward) either before or after the QRS complex
QRS complex and T wave usually normal

Treatment: Monitor vital signs. If vital signs and patient are stable, treat underlying cause: myocardial infarction, congestive heart failure, acidosis, hyperkalemia
Continued on following page

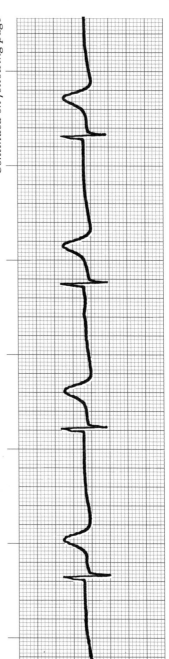

Questions:

Establish intravenous access; prepare pacemaker

AMPLER/PQRST. Medications?

Next Step:

Carefully monitor vital signs and mental status. Keep pacemaker and medications nearby

NORMAL SINUS RHYTHM WITH RATE OF 100 BEATS PER MINUTE

Name: Normal sinus rhythm (regular sinus rhythm)

Description: 60–100 beats per minute
Each complex is complete: P wave, QRS complex, T wave
No untoward, wide, bizarre, ectopic, early, late, or different-looking complexes
All intervals within normal limits

Treatment: Monitor vital signs; check blood pressure

Questions: AMPLER

Next Step: Monitor patient's condition

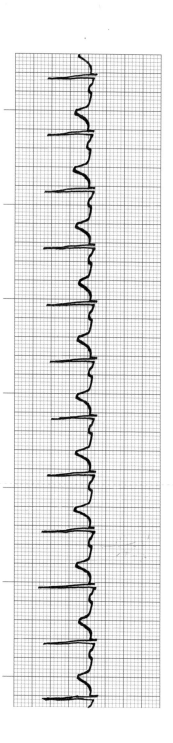

Glossary

....

ABC. The abbreviation for airway, breathing, circulation. The first three steps of basic life support.

absolute refractory. The early phase of cardiac repolarization in which the heart muscle cannot be stimulated to depolarize.

acidosis. A disturbance in the acid-base balance of the body, an excess of acid.

ACLS. Advanced Cardiac Life Support. A series of protocols and standards set by the American Heart Association for the resuscitation and treatment of cardiac patients.

agonal rhythm. Cardiac rhythm seen just before asystole, associated with infrequent wide QRS complexes and no cardiac output or pulse.

AMI. acute myocardial infarction, a heart attack.

AMPLER. Allergies, medications, past history, last meal, events leading to, risk factors. A memory system for patient history.

anatomical position. The position of a patient who is upright, facing forward, hands by the sides with palms facing forward.

antiarrhythmic drug. Any drug given to prevent or terminate cardiac dysrhythmias.

APE. acute pulmonary edema; left-sided congestive heart failure.

apical pulse. A pulse taken by listening over the apical portion of the heart for 60 seconds.

arrhythmia. Any deviation from the normal rhythm of the heart.

atria. The two top chambers of the heart.

atrial depolarization. Electrical process resulting in atrial contraction, represented by the P wave on the ECG.

atrial fibrillation. A dysrhythmia characterized by multiple rapid ectopic atrial foci and an irregular ventricular response.

atrial flutter. A dysrhythmia characterized by a single, rapid, ectopic atrial focus resulting in a sawtooth pattern to the ECG, as the AV node conducts impulses in a set pattern, e.g., 3:1, 4:1.

atropine. A drug used to increase the speed of the heart by blocking the parasympathetic nervous system.

AV node. Atrioventricular node. Portion of the cardiac conduction system that conducts impulses from the atria.

baseline. Isoelectric line of the ECG.

blocked impulse. An electrical impulse that is stopped or slowed at a certain point and not conducted further through the system.

b/p. Blood pressure.

bpm. Beats per minute.

brady-. Prefix meaning slow.

bradycardia. Slow heart rate, under 60 beats per minute.

bundle branches. The portion of the conduction system of the heart that conducts impulses from the bundle of His to the Purkinje fibers and works to contract the ventricles.

bundle of His. The portion of the conduction system of the heart that conducts impulses from the AV node to the bundle branches and works to contract the ventricles.

CaCl. Calcium chloride.

cardia(o)-. Prefix pertaining to the heart.

cardiac arrest. The sudden cessation of cardiac activity.

cardiac cycle. The period from one cardiac contraction to the next.

cardiac output. Stroke volume × heart rate.

cardioversion. Application of a synchronized electrical current to restore the heart's conduction system to a normal rhythm or function.

CHF. Congestive heart failure. Failure of adequate ventricular function, which results in the backup of blood or fluid.

coarse V-fib. The uncoordinated beating of many weak ectopic ventricular foci, which results in a squiggly line on the ECG. Illustrates possibly viable electrical activity in the heart.

code. A signal used to summon a team of medical professionals trained to administer CPR/ACLS to a patient in cardiac arrest.

compensatory pause. A change in the R-R interval that follows a premature or delayed beat and restores the original rhythm.

complexes. Waveform made on the ECG tracing, representing electrical conduction throughout the heart. Can refer to the QRS *complex* (contraction of the ventricles) or the entire sequence (P-QRS-T) as in the number of *complexes* in 1 minute.

conduction. The ability of the electrical system of the heart to transmit impulses from cell to cell.

contraction. The shortening of a muscle, in this case the heart.

coronary arteries. The arteries that supply blood to the heart muscle.

CPR. Cardiopulmonary resuscitation. Ventilation combined with external chest compressions provided to patients in cardiac arrest.

defib pads/paddles. Large pads or paddles attached to a defibrillator, used to deliver an electrical shock to a patient.

defibrillation. Application of an unsynchronized electrical shock in an effort to restore a normal cardiac rhythm.

defibrillator. A device that is used to deliver strong electrical current to restore regular rhythms from uncoordinated ones.

deflection. The direction of a complex on the ECG in relation to the isoelectric line. Deflected upward (above) or downward (below) relative to the baseline.

depolarization. The conduction of an impulse through the myocardium when the cells go from negatively charged to positively charged.

diastolic. Pertaining to the relaxation phase of the heart.

digoxin. Lanoxin, a medication given to regulate a rapid heart rate.

dropped beats. Cardiac impulses created by a pacemaker but not conducted through the electrical system. They usually appear as a lone P wave on the ECG strip not followed by a QRS complex or a T wave.

drug toxicity. Having in excess of the therapeutic level of a medication in the blood.

ECG. Electrocardiogram, also known as EKG. The electrical activity of the heart displayed on a screen or recorded on paper.

ectopic. Located away from a normal position. For instance, an ectopic complex is an impulse generated from cells outside the usual pacemaker sites.

Einthoven. Inventor of the ECG machine.

EKG. Electrocardiogram, also known as ECG; see **ECG**.

electrodes. Small pads placed on the chest wall that convert the electrical activity of the heart to a dynamic display on a monitor.

f waves. The fibrillatory waves of atrial fibrillation. Frequent irregular waves caused by multiple weak ectopic foci.

F waves. Flutter waves of atrial flutter. The repetitive, rapid, regular beating of one irritable focus in the atrium characterized by a sawtooth pattern on ECG.

fever. A temperature above 98.6° F or 37° C.

focus. One cell generating electrical activity that originates outside a usual pacemaker site. (Plural: foci.)

hemodynamic. The force involved in circulating the blood through the body.

hyperkalemia. Excessive amount of potassium in the blood.

hypotension. Low blood pressure.

hypoxia. Diminished amount of oxygen in the tissues, usually the result of inadequate respirations.

Inderal. Propranolol, a beta blocker used to slow the heart rate and control irregular rhythms.

intrinsic. Inherent or inborn, from within.

intubate. Insert a tube into the trachea to secure an airway.

irregular. When the measure of the R-R interval varies in an ECG rhythm.

ischemia. Muscle tissue damaged from lack of oxygen in the heart; the damaged part of the heart muscle does not respond to electrical stimuli in the same way healthy muscle does, resulting in arrhythmias.

IV. Intravenous.

junctional impulses. Impulses originating in the AV node, or the AV junction.

large box. On the ECG paper, one large box is made up of five small boxes and is equivalent to 0.20 second.

lidocaine. An antiarrhythmic medication given to reduce ectopic activity.

MI. Myocardial infarction.

mm. Millimeter.

monitor. The screen on which ECG rhythms are viewed.

multifocal. Originating from more than one ectopic pacemaker site.

myocardium. The muscle cells of the heart.

nodal. Originating in the AV node.

node. The name of a part of the electrical conduction system of the heart; i.e., SA node, AV node.

P wave. The graphic representation of the depolarization of the atria on the ECG.

PAC. Premature atrial contraction.

paced rhythm. A cardiac rhythm created by an artificial pacemaker placed in the heart.

pacemaker. (1) Specialized tissue within the heart that initiates electrical activity and causes the heart to contract. (2) A battery-powered device, placed in the heart, designed to sense a decrease in cardiac activity and create electrical activity causing the heart to contract in the absence of intrinsic pacemaker activity.

paroxysmal. Sudden and intense occurrence of symptoms.

PQRST. (1) Alphabetical name of the waves of the ECG developed by Einthoven. (2) Acronym for provokes, quality, radiation, severity, time. A memory system for assessing chest pain.

P-R interval. The interval measured from the beginning of the P wave to the beginning of the R wave; should be no more than 0.12–0.20 second or three to five small boxes and represents the path of the impulse through the atria and AV junction.

precordial thump. Procedure used for witnessed cardiac arrest in which the rescuer uses a closed fist to strike a patient over the sternum in an effort to restore cardiac activity.

premature. Arriving earlier than expected.

primary pacemaker. SA node of the heart; located highest in the heart and having the fastest intrinsic firing rate.

Pt. Patient.

Purkinje fibers. Portion of the heart's conduction system that helps to contract the ventricles.

PVC. Premature ventricular contraction.

QRS complex. The graphic representation of the depolarization of the ventricles on ECG.

quinidine. An antiarrhythmic medication used to slow conduction.

ratio. Conduction of impulses in a pattern, e.g., 3:1, 4:1, 5:1.

refractory. The repolarization stage of the heart.

regular. A constant R-R interval throughout a rhythm strip.

relative refractory. The period of time during repolarization when the heart is still susceptible to strong stimulus.

repolarization. Relaxation phase of the myocardium.

retrograde. Backward conduction of an impulse, upward through the heart instead of downward.

r/o. Rule out.

R-R interval. The measured distance between two R waves. This distance should be constant throughout the rhythm strip for the rhythm to be considered regular.

r/t. Related to.

SA node. Sinoatrial node, the primary pacemaker of the heart. Highest in location, and fastest in intrinsic firing rate.

septum. Cartilage tissue that divides the heart into left and right halves.

shock. Inadequate tissue perfusion.

sign. Clinical indicator that you can see or measure.

sinus. Normal.

sinus rhythm. Normal, regular cardiac rhythm.

small box. Representation on ECG paper of 0.04 second.

S/S. Signs and symptoms.

sternum. The bone that lies in the center of the chest, the breastbone.

symptom. Clinical indicator that the patient reports. See **sign**.

symptomatic. Showing clinical indicators of a condition; e.g., *symptomatic bradycardia* is a slow heartbeat accompanied by dizziness and weakness.

syncope. Fainting.

systole. The part of the cardiac cycle that represents the heart contracting and pushing blood out of the lungs and body.

T wave. The waveform on the ECG that represents the repolarization of the ventricles of the heart.

tachy-. Prefix meaning fast.

tachycardia. A fast heart rate, above 100 beats per minute.

tx. Treatment.

uncoordinated. Cells in the heart firing electrical activity at different times, resulting in no true contraction of the heart muscle. The heart looks like a "bag of worms."

unifocal. Electrical activity originating from one irritable cell in the heart, not a primary pacemaker.

untoward. Unexpected.

vagal maneuvers. Physical actions designed to stimulate the vagus nerve and slow down rapid heart rates, such as bearing down as if to have a bowel movement, carotid sinus massage or pressing on both eyes.

vagal tone. Pertaining to innervation of the 10th cranial nerve, the vagus nerve, which is the chief mediator of the parasympathetic nervous system. Stimulation of this nerve slows down heart rate.

vasovagal. Usually used to refer to a syndrome in which a patient accidentally stimulates the vagus nerve, e.g., by bearing down to have a bowel movement, resulting in a slowed heart rate and an episode of syncope.

ventricles. The two lower chambers of the heart.

ventricular fibrillation. Weak, rapid, disorganized discharge of multiple ventricular ectopic foci resulting in a squiggly line on the ECG. It may appear coarse or fine.

v/s. Vital signs.